GREAT HAIR

Elegant Styles for Every Occasion

By

Davis Biton

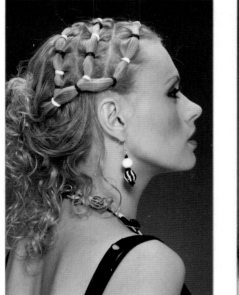
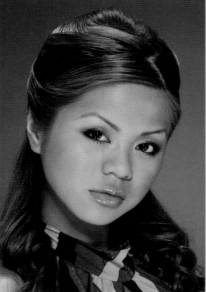
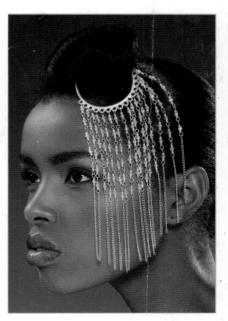

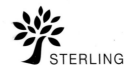

STERLING

New York / London
www.sterlingpublishing.com

Designed by Eddie Goldfine
Edited by Shoshana Brickman
Photography by Ohad Romano
Layout by Gala Pre Press Ltd.

STERLING and the distinctive Sterling logo are registered trademarks of Sterling Publishing Co., Inc.

Library of Congress Cataloging-in-Publication Data

Biton, Davis.
 Great hair : elegant styles for every occasion / Davis Biton.
    p. cm.
 Includes index.
 ISBN-13: 978-1-4027-4736-6
 ISBN-10: 1-4027-4736-5
 1. Hairdressing. 2. Hairstyles. I. Title.

TT972.B49 2007
646.7'24--dc22

                                    2007020495

10 9 8 7 6 5

Published by Sterling Publishing Co., Inc.
387 Park Avenue South, New York, NY 10016
Penn Publishing Ltd.
1 Yehuda Halevi St., Tel Aviv, Israel 65135
© 2007 by Penn Publishing Ltd.
Distributed in Canada by Sterling Publishing
C/o Canadian Manda Group, 165 Dufferin Street
Toronto, Ontario, Canada M6K 3H6
Distributed in the United Kingdom by GMC Distribution Services
Castle Place, 166 High Street, Lewes, East Sussex, England BN7 1XU
Distributed in Australia by Capricorn Link (Australia) Pty. Ltd.
P.O. Box 704, Windsor, NSW 2756, Australia

Sterling ISBN-13: 978-1-4027-4736-6
       ISBN-10: 1-4027-4736-5

For information about custom editions, special sales, premium and corporate purchases, please contact Sterling Special Sales Department at 800-805-5489 or specialsales@sterlingpub.com.

CONTENTS

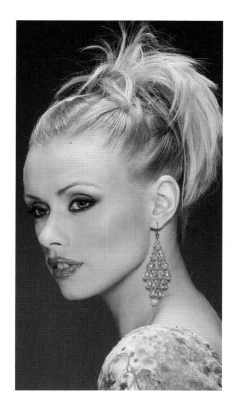

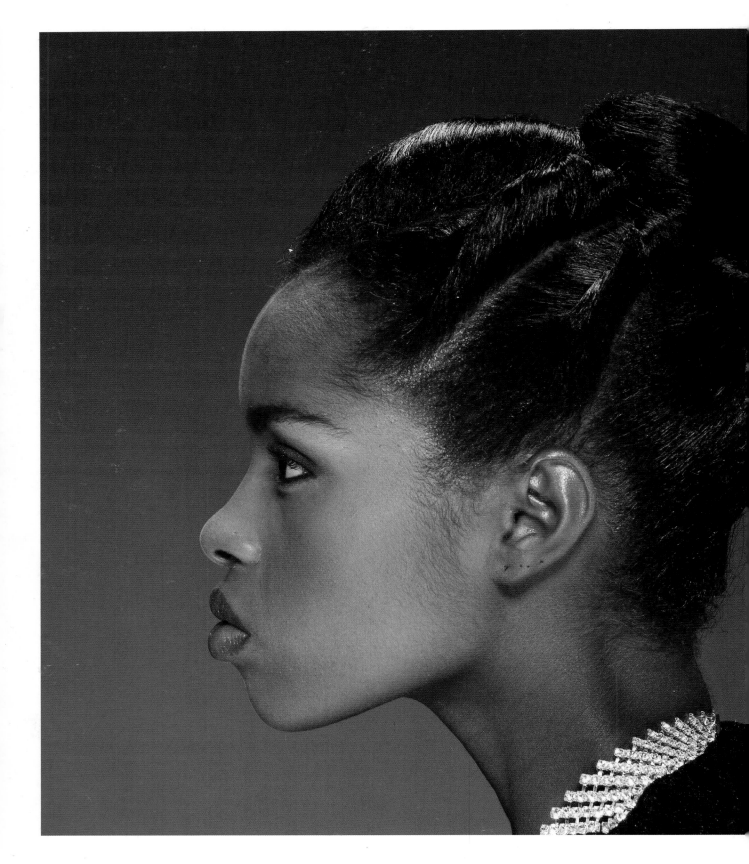

INTRODUCTION

Going to a hairstylist before every special occasion can be expensive and time-consuming. Why not create your own fabulous hairstyle at home? Not only is it much less expensive than going to a stylist, it also means you can do your hair according to your schedule, not someone else's!

In *Great Hair: Elegant Styles for Every Occasion*, you'll find hairstyles for every type of hair, and for any occasion. There are styles for long hair and short hair; styles for curly hair and straight hair. If you like integrating hair extensions or accessories, you'll find a few hairstyles that use these, too.

As for occasions, there are options suitable for every affair. Elegant styles that are perfect for weddings or fancy parties; funky designs that are ideal for an evening of dinner and dancing. Techniques for making carefree braids, romantic curls, exotic loops, and subtle waves are included as well.

Just select the occasion, and choose a hairstyle to match. Better still, make an occasion out of a new hairstyle!

About the Author

Davis Biton is a leading international hairstyling artist. The creative force behind the *Davis* brand of hair care products, Davis runs a vibrant salon, operates a distinguished hair academy, and travels the world participating in professional exhibitions. Davis has published several books on hair design, including the three-volume series *Hair Creation Gallery* and the multi-volume French-English series *The Art of Dressing Hair*.

ESSENTIAL SUPPLIES AND TIPS

You'll need a few basic supplies for completing the hairstyles in this book. These can be found in hair salons, beauty supply shops, and department stores. Of course, the Internet has a large variety of sites for ordering online.

Essential Supplies

Blow dryer You'll need one of these to dry hair before you start your hairstyle. In many cases, you'll blow dry hair as you style it and to dry spray and mousse.

Bobby pins These small pins are used to secure hair closely on the head. A bobby pin is made of a single bent wire. One side of the pin is straight and the other side is kinked. Both sides touch each other.

Clips Metal and plastic clips of various sizes are used to hold one section of hair to the side while another section is being styled.

Curling iron This is essential for making ringlets. Curling irons come in various sizes, so choose the one you use according to the size of curls you want.

Diffuser This adds volume to curly hair, and really brings out the curls.

Elastic bands These are used to secure ponytails and braids. Choose elastic bands that are gentle on your hair and don't rip it. Although the color may be important in some hairstyles, an elastic band is often concealed by wrapping a lock of hair around it.

Finishing spray Spray this after you have finished styling the hair to hold the style. Spray while styling for particularly high styles.

Hair accessories These are used in a number of hairstyles. They range from decorated hairpins to beaded hairnets, ribbons, and pieces of jewelry.

Hair extensions These additions, made from natural or synthetic hair, may be long or short, curly or straight. Use a hair extension that matches your natural color, or integrate one that contrasts for a more dramatic effect. Hair extensions can be used over and over again, just be sure to care for them properly.

Hair straightener This iron-like device is used to flatten hair, and hold a tight roll in place.

Hairpins These small pins are used to secure hair on the head. A hairpin is made with a single bent wire. Both sides of the wire are kinked and they do not touch each other.

Holding spray Spray this onto hair as you sculpt it to make hair flexible while holding a style. Holding spray should not make the hair too stiff to shape.

Needle and thread A number of hairstyles require the use of a blunt needle and thick thread, either for attaching a hair extension or for securing hair in place. Be sure to use a blunt needle when sewing, and ask a friend for help if necessary. Also, consider the thread you select in advance. Do you want it to blend into your hair or stand out?

Styling cream Apply this generously to dry hair to

make it softer and easier to work with. It is especially important when blow drying hair, as extra heat can damage already dry hair.

Rollers There are various types of rollers on the market. Select the size of the rollers according to the size of curl you prefer.

Round brush Also known as radial brushes, these brushes can be used to add curls when blow drying hair, and to add volume and body.

Sponge This is integrated into hair to add structure and volume.

Styling gel This adds moisture to dry hair, and helps you sculpt a style and hold it.

Styling mousse Work this into wet hair before styling it. Use strong styling mousse before setting hair in rollers.

Tail comb These combs, also called rattail combs, have teeth at one end and a fine point at the other end. Use the teeth for backcombing hair; use the fine point for making parts, or for holding hair in place while styling. Hairstyles that have many loops and twists may require you to use several tail combs.

Wide tooth comb Use this to separate locks of hair.

Tips

Gathering supplies Prepare yourself before you start a hairstyle. Make sure you have all the elastic bands, clips, tail combs, and hairpins you'll need. You'll also want to have enough hair spray and styling mousse on hand.

Preparing the hair
Start each of these hairstyles with clean, tangle-free hair. Use a gentle brush to make sure there are no tangles before you start.

Styling with a friend
In some cases, you may want to have a friend help you style the hair, either by inviting her to do the hairstyle for you, by practicing on her first, or by having her help out with some trickier aspects of the design.

Making parts
To make a tidy hairstyle, you have to start with a tidy base. This means making parts that are smooth and straight. Use a tail comb to make parts, be patient, and be precise. The result is worth it.

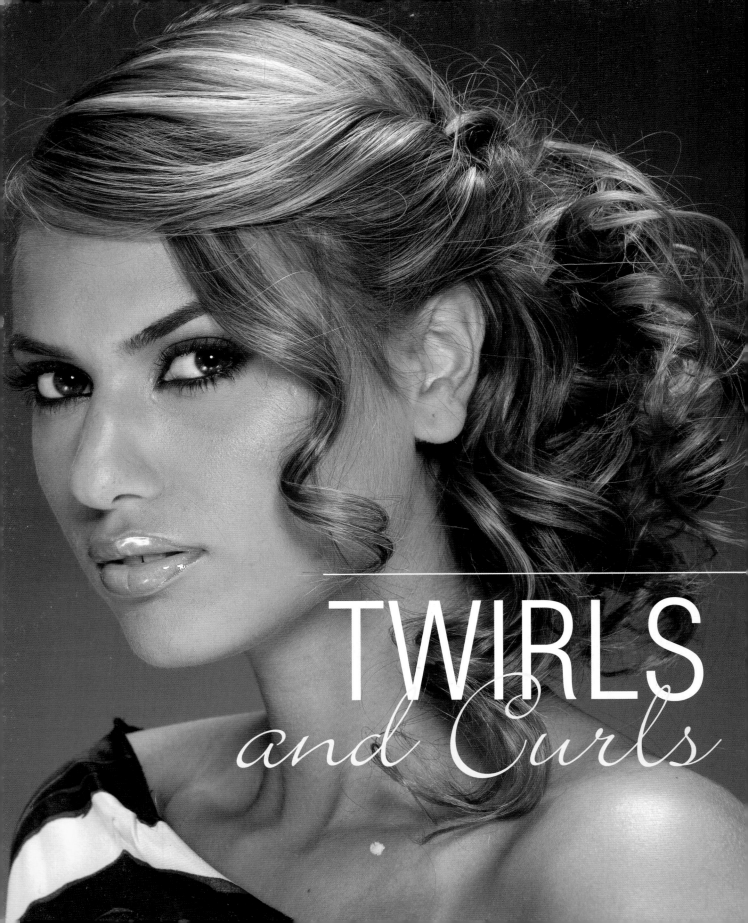

TWIRLS
and Curls

1

1. Wash and blow dry hair. Curl the hair into loose ringlets with a curling iron.

2. Let hair cool a few minutes, then separate each ringlet into five locks.

3. Divide the hair into front and back sections with a part that extends from ear to ear over the crown. Divide the front section with a right side part. Divide the back section into two sections. Divide one of the back sections into top and bottom sections.

4. Twist the top and bottom sections together to form a rope.

Create a playful, carefree look by drawing the hair away from the face and allowing the locks to cascade loosely down the back.

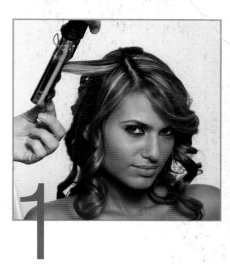

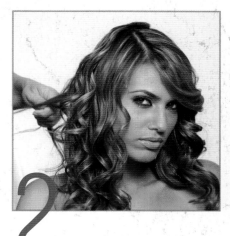

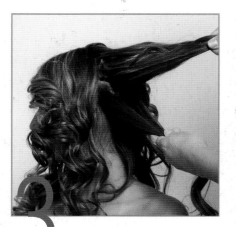

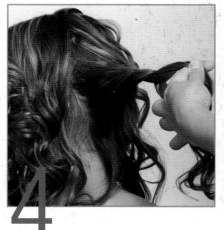

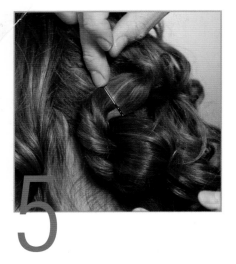

5

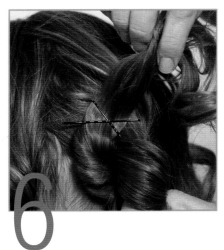

6

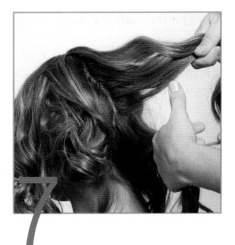

7

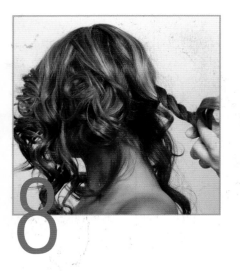

8

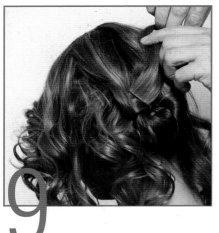

9

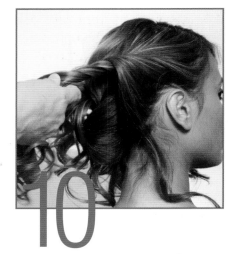

10

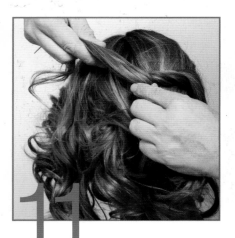

11

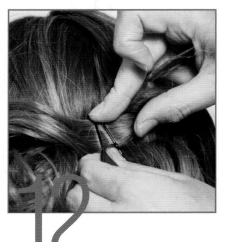

12

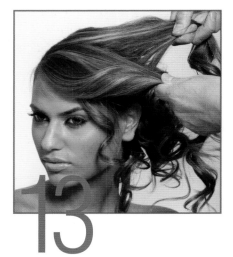

13

5. Coil the rope inwards.

6. Secure the coil with an X of bobby pins, leaving the ends loose.

7. Divide the other section of hair at the back into top and bottom sections.

8. Twist the sections together to form a rope.

9. Coil the rope and secure with an X of bobby pins.

10. Move to the front hair. Divide the hair on the right side of the part into two sections and twist the sections to form a rope.

11. Draw the rope around the back of the head, towards the X of bobby pins on the right side.

12. Secure with pins close to the X of pins.

13. Move to the remaining section of hair at the front. Divide the hair into front and back sections. Draw out a lock of hair to fall gently on the face.

14. Twist the sections to form a rope.

15. Draw the rope around the back of the head and secure close to the X of pins.

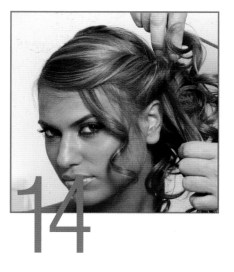

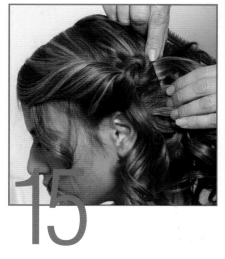

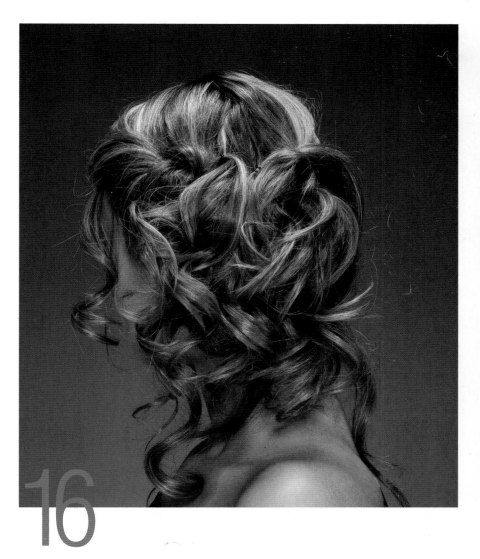

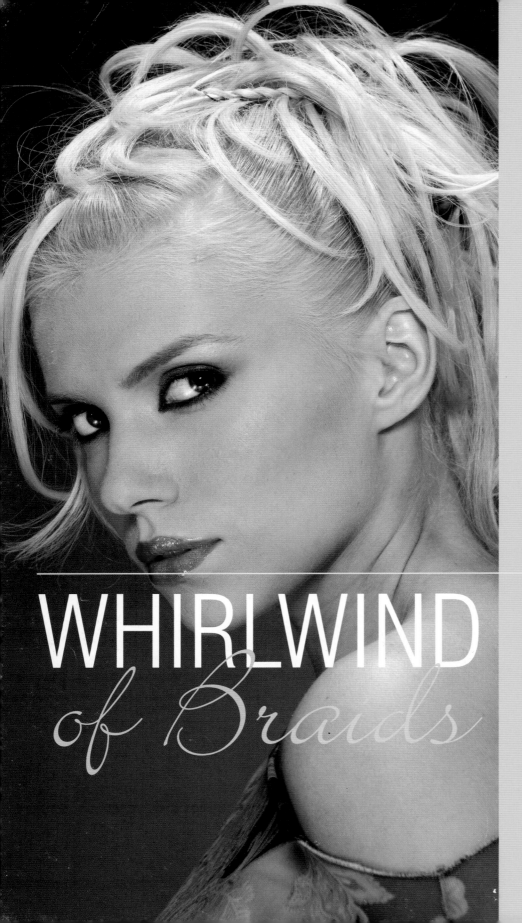

WHIRLWIND
of Braids

2

Braids get a twist—literally—with this unusual design. It features several braids that are wrapped around the back of the head. Each braid has a few drawn-out strands, creating a windswept appearance.

1. Wash and blow dry hair straight. Gather the hair at the top with a large clip. Make a part that extends from the outer edge of each eyebrow around the back of the head and gather the hair above this part in a ponytail at the back.

2. Make four more ponytails at the back of the head, each of them the same size and directly below the first ponytail.

3. Begin by plaiting a braid in the bottom ponytail.

4. Draw out a few strands of hair with every second plait to give the braid a windswept appearance.

5. Follow the same technique to make a similar braid in the second ponytail from the bottom.

6. Divide the hair in the third ponytail from the bottom into two sections. Make a windswept braid in each section. Repeat to plait two windswept braids in the two remaining ponytails.

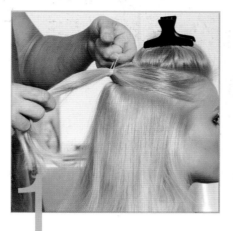

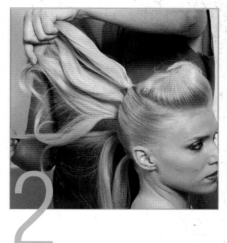

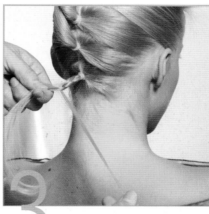

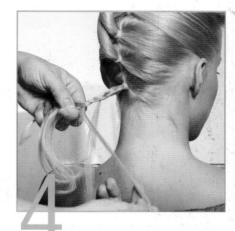

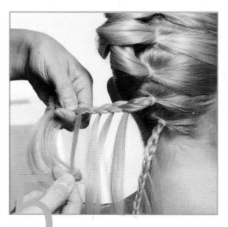

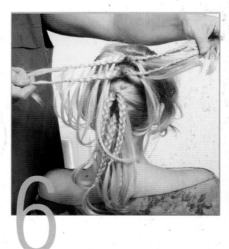

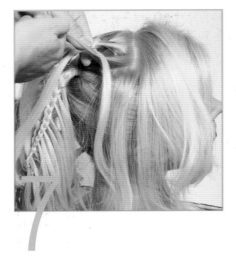

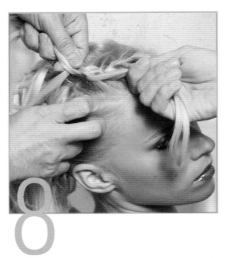

7. Release the hair from the clip at the top and divide the hair into front and back sections. Begin plaiting a braid with the hair in the back section.

8. Continue the braid, drawing out a few strands of hair with every second plait to make a windswept braid.

9. Repeat with the hair in the front section, starting with a French braid, then continuing to make a windswept braid.

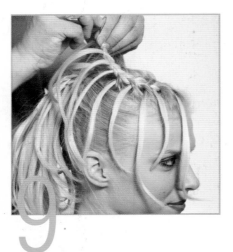

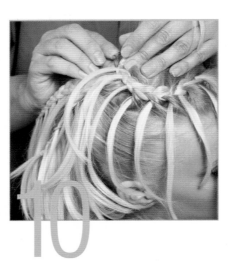

10. Wrap the bottom braid around the front and secure at the back of the head, just above the top ponytail.

11. Draw the braid from the back section around to the front and secure at the top of the ponytail.

12. Continue wrapping the braids around the front of the head, working your way towards the nape of the neck, and pinning each braid above the previous braid to create a cascade of windswept braids.

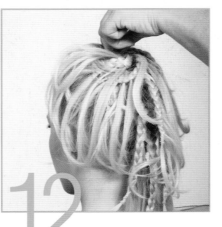

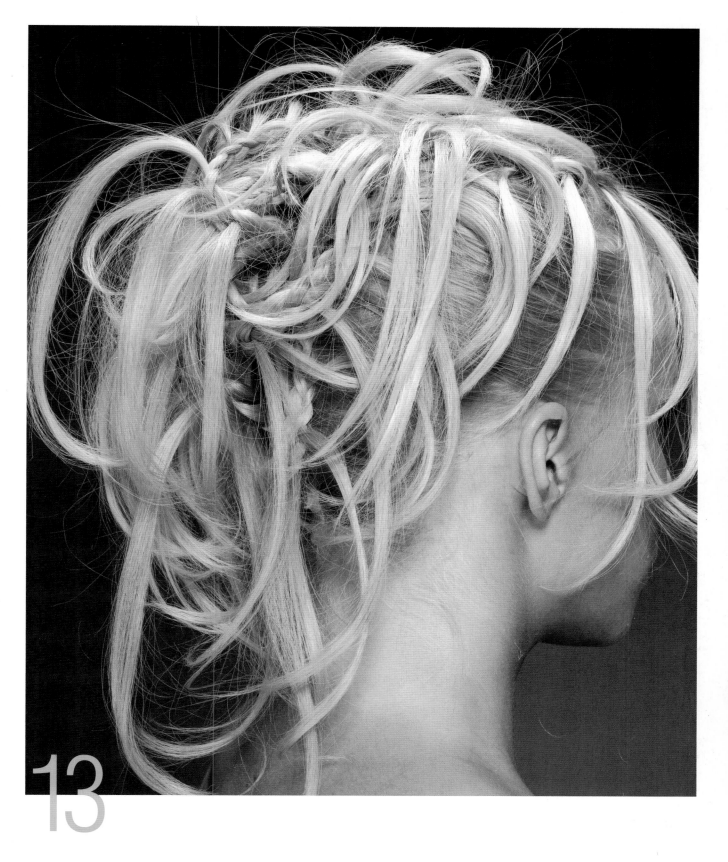

13

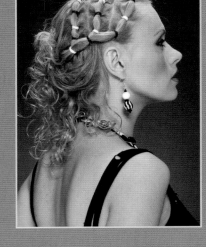

CHECKERBOARD

Braids

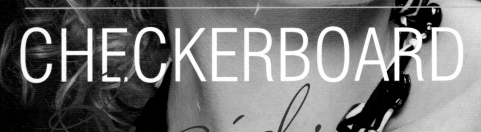

Use black and white elastic bands to make a checkerboard pattern with this hairstyle. Perfect for topping off a tuxedo-style pantsuit.

3

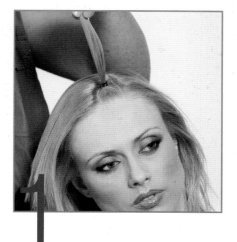

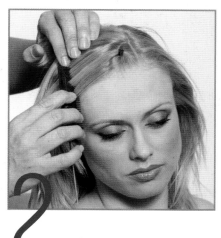

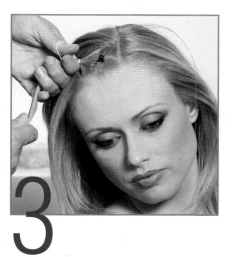

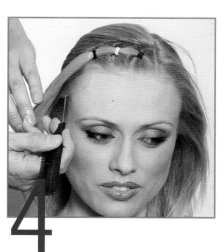

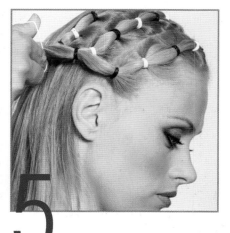

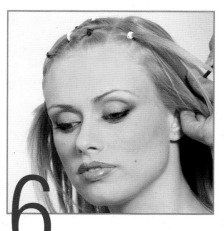

1. Wash and blow dry hair straight. Make a left side part from the brow to the crown. Gather hair from a 1-inch section at the brow and to the right of the part in a ponytail near the roots.

2. Brush the ponytail to the right, integrating it into the loose hair.

3. Gather hair from a similar section to the right of the first ponytail and make a ponytail that includes the first ponytail. Use a different color elastic band to secure the second ponytail.

4. Continue linking ponytails to make a braid of ponytails that ends at the right ear. Alternate the color of the elastic bands to make a checkerboard effect.

5. Repeat the technique to make two more ponytail braids behind the first one. Join all three ponytail braids with an elastic band.

6. Repeat the same technique on the left side of the part to make three ponytail braids.

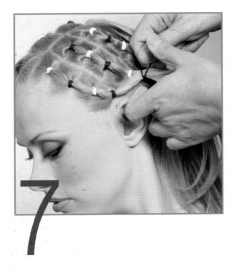 **7**

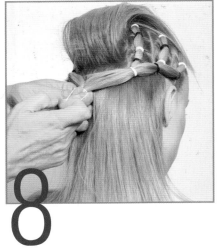 **8**

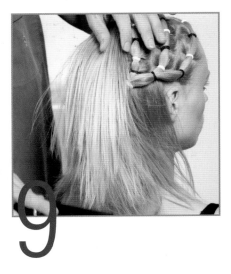 **9**

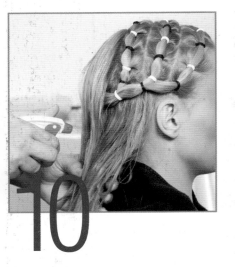 **10**

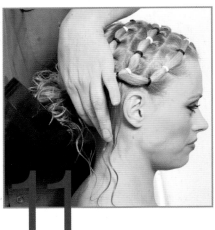 **11**

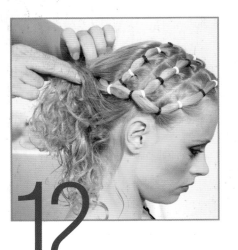 **12**

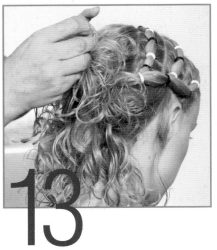 **13**

7. Join the three ponytail braids with an elastic band.

8. Make a part along the back of the head, at the line where the two ponytail braids end. Brush the hair above the part upwards and draw the ponytail braids together in a ponytail at the back.

9. Brush down the hair from above the part to cover the ponytail at the back.

10. Wet the loose hair with liquid spray or styling mousse.

11. Blow dry the loose hair with a diffuser.

12. Lift the loose hair on the right and left sides of the head upwards.

13. Secure with pins at the back.

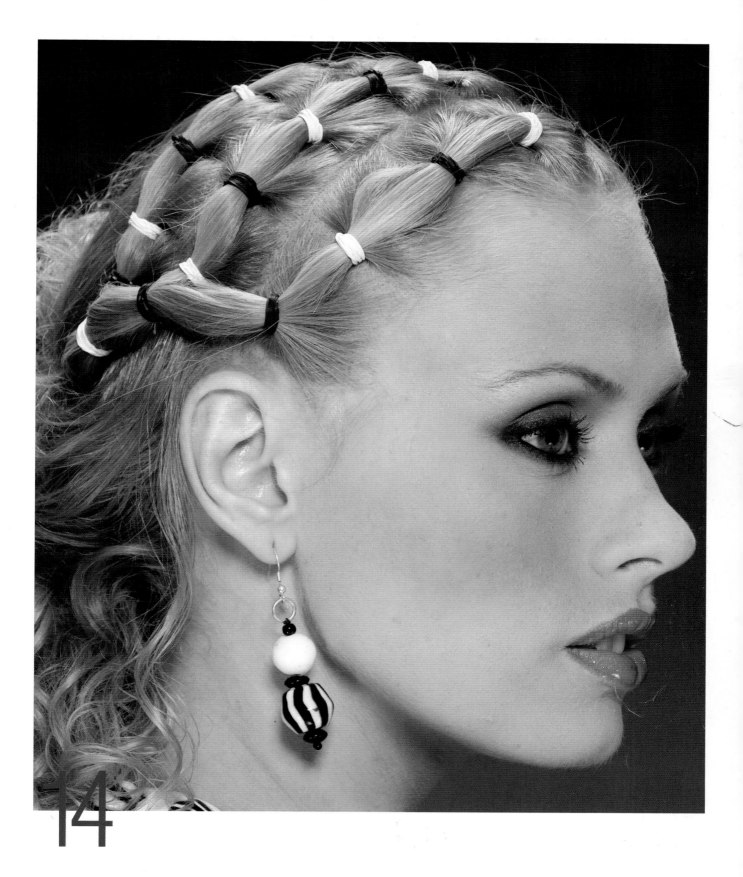

14

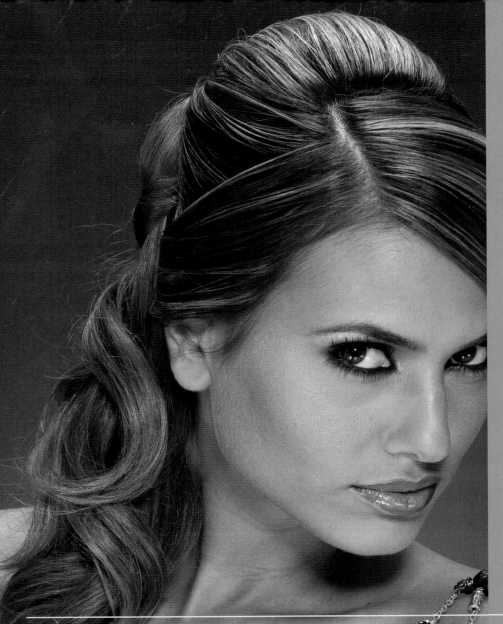

4

CASCADING
Waterfall

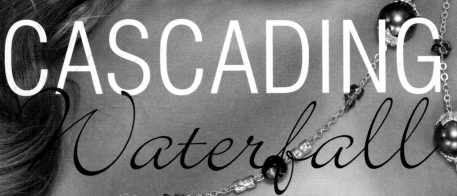

Long hair cascades like a flowing waterfall in this style. The top features eddying twirls; the bottom cascades loosely down the back.

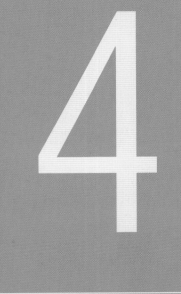

1. Wash and blow dry hair. Curl the hair into loose ringlets with a curling iron.

2. Make a right side part from the brow to the crown. Backcomb the hair at the crown.

3. Backcomb a round section of hair at the crown.

4. Brush the front hair at the middle of the head over the backcombed section. Secure with a seam of pins at the back of the head.

5. Divide the front hair on the right side of the part into front and back sections. Brush the back section into a flat strip and draw it backwards towards the seam of pins.

6. Wrap the hair over the seam of pins to conceal it and secure on the left side.

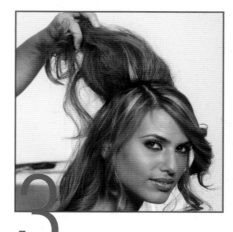

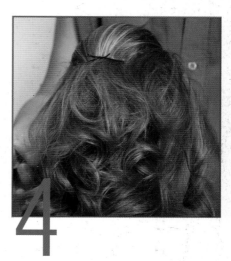

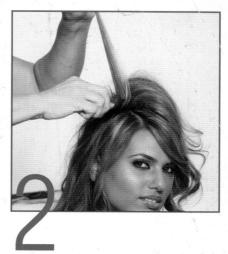

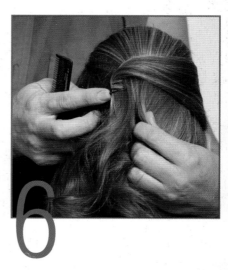

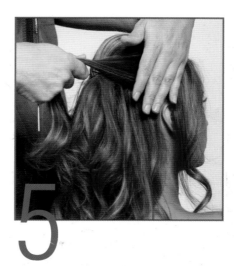

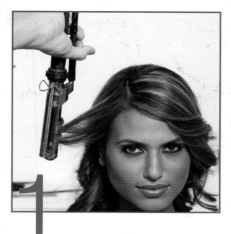

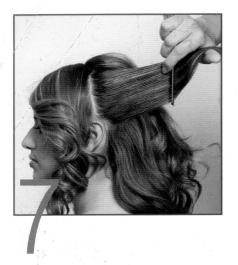

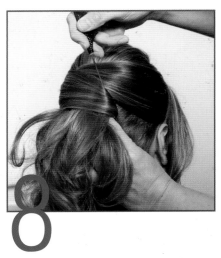

7. Divide the front hair on the left side of the part into front and back sections. Brush the back section into a flat strip and draw backwards.

8. Wrap this section of hair diagonally downwards over the seam of pins.

9. Secure with a bobby pin under the seam of pins.

10. Brush the remaining section of hair on the front right side backwards and downwards. Secure at the back under the seam of pins.

11. Brush the remaining section of hair on the front left side into a flat strip.

12. Secure at the back, under the hair that was pinned previously.

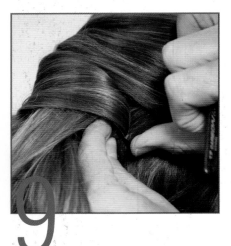

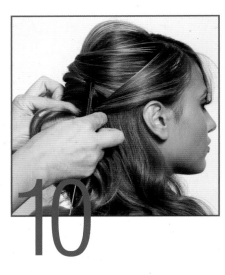

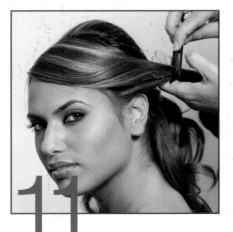

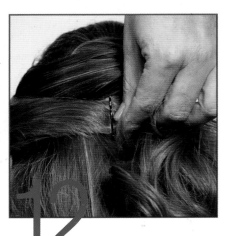

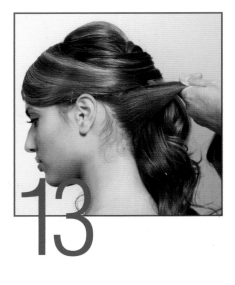

13. Take a section of hair from behind the left ear and brush upwards and over towards the right side.

14. Secure with a pin over the hair that was pinned previously.

15. Draw a lock of hair from the back and brush into a flat strip. Coil upwards into a flat Figure 6 and secure with a pin at the back.

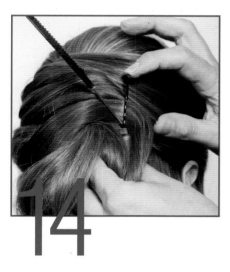

14

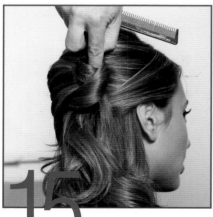

15

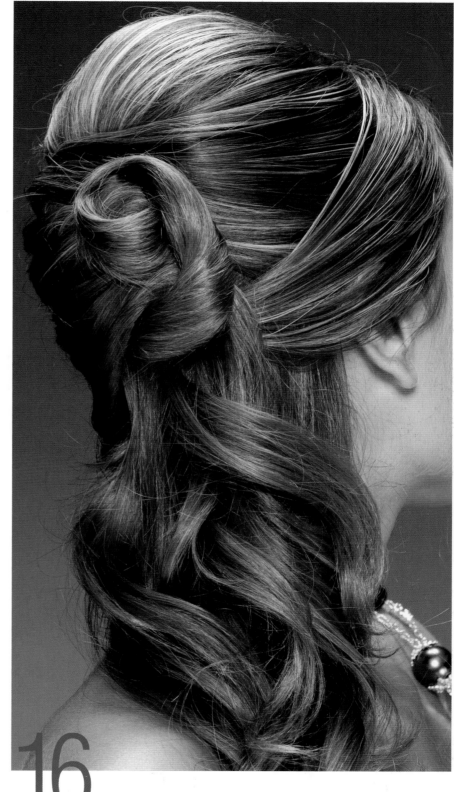

16

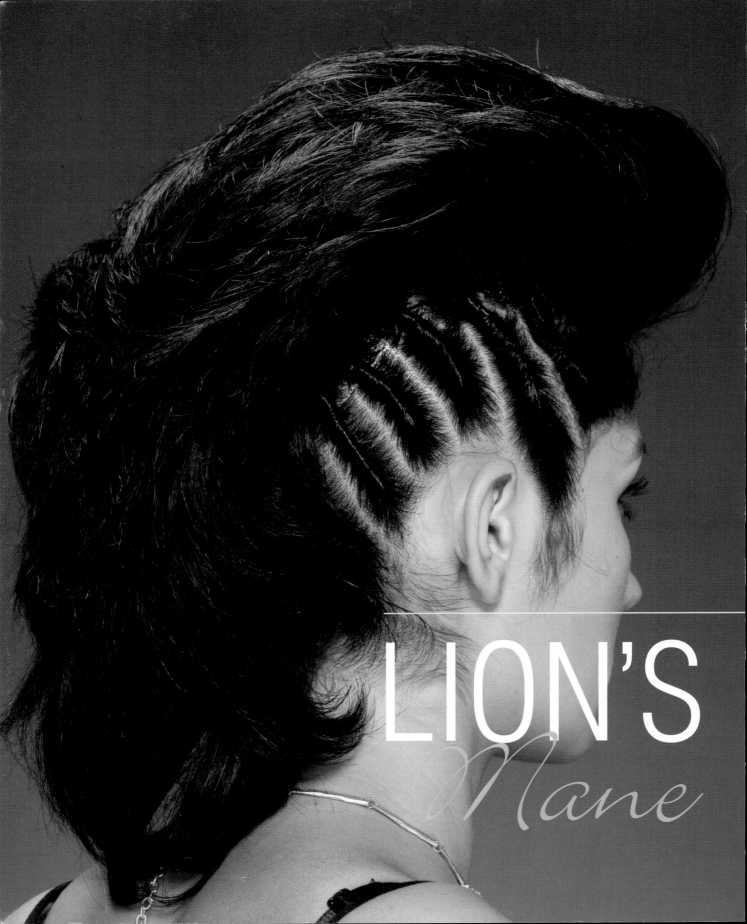

LION'S
Mane

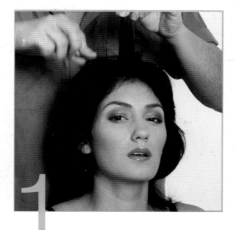

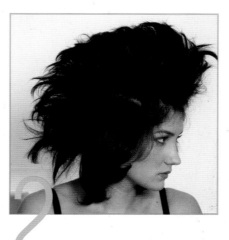

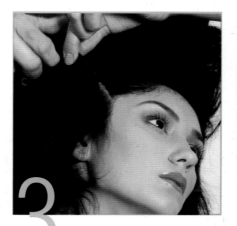

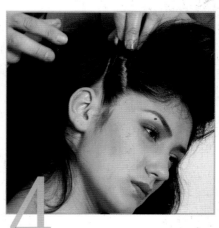

5

There is nothing subtle about this style. Roaring with personality and presence, it is a perfect design for any occasion that merits a real statement.

1. Wash and blow dry hair upwards. Backcomb the bangs.

2. Backcomb the hair behind, all the way from brow to the nape of the neck.

3. Move to the right side of the head. Gather a lock of hair at the front and mist with holding spray. Twist the lock close to the roots and upwards, towards the backcombed hair at the top. Secure with a hairpin.

4. Twist another lock of hair behind the first one that is equal in width. Secure below the backcombed hair with a hairpin.

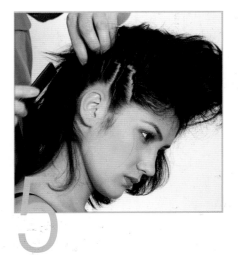

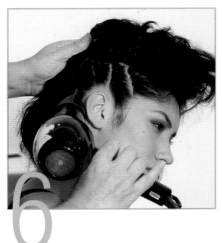

5. Repeat all the way along the right side of the head until the nape of the neck. Repeat on the left side as well.

6. Mist with holding spray and blow dry.

7. Using a blunt needle and thick thread, sew the twisted locks in place. Start at the front, drawing the thread under the pins at the top of each coiled strip as you work your way backwards.

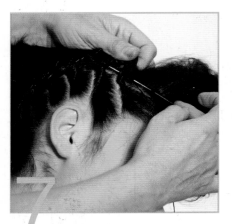

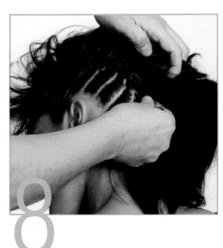

8. Remove the hairpins after the spray has dried.

9. Mist with finishing spray.

10. Blow dry to secure. Repeat on the other side.

11. Use a wide tooth comb to style the hair at the top so that it flows gently backwards.

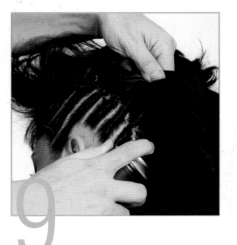

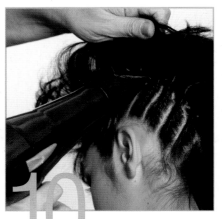

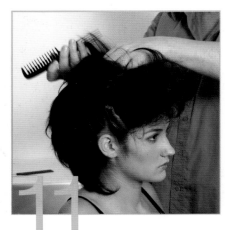

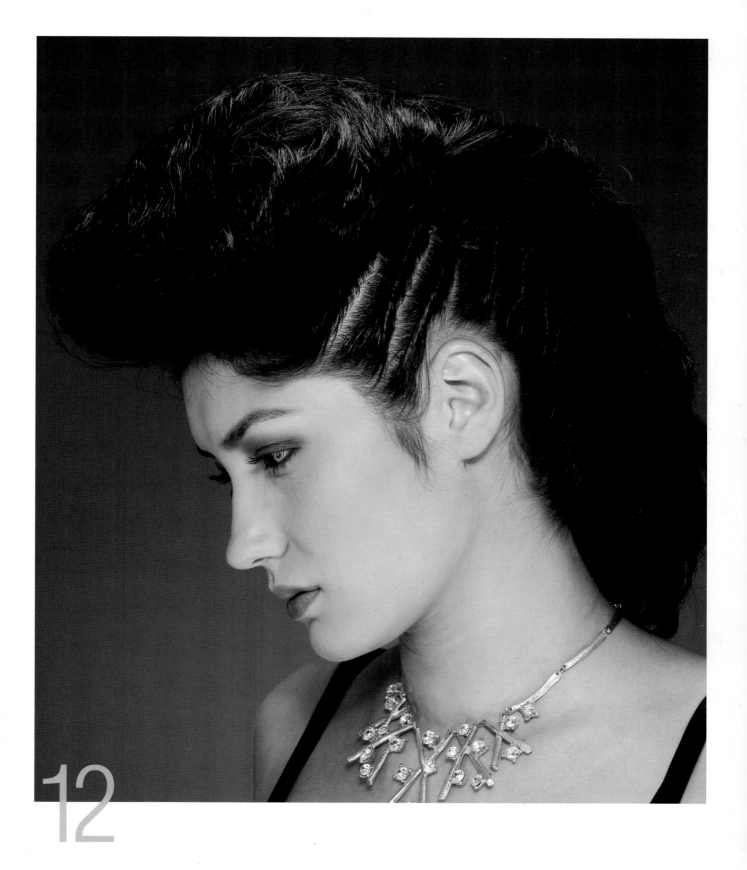

12

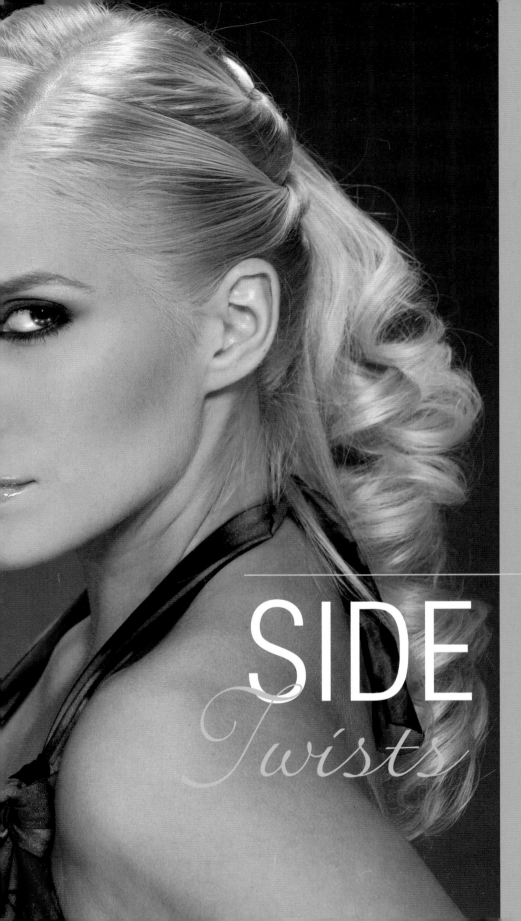

SIDE
Twists

6

Graceful twists on either side of the face make an elegantly feminine frame. This style is light and romantic—ideal for a springtime wedding.

1. Wash and blow dry hair wavy, running fingers through the hair to loosen the waves. Make a left side part from the brow to the crown.

2. Make a rectangular part at the back that extends from the crown to the nape of the neck. Gather the hair on the right and left sides of the part in clips.

3. Backcomb the hair at the top of the rectangular section.

4. Backcomb all of the hair in this section to make a spongy base that extends to the nape of the neck.

5. Make a diagonal part on the left side of the head, just above the spongy base. Gather the hair in this section and twist gently towards the spongy base.

6. Secure the hair with hairpins to the spongy base.

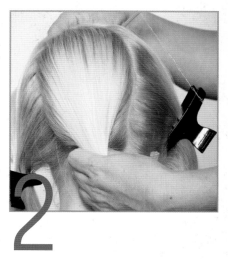

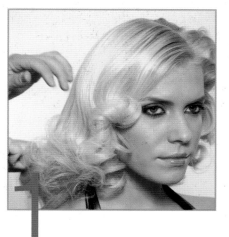

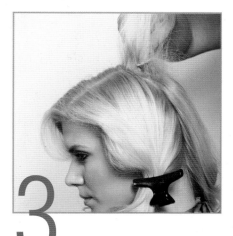

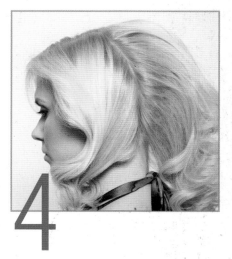

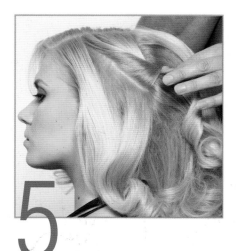

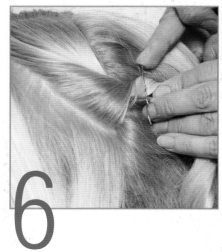

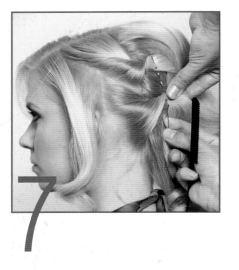

7

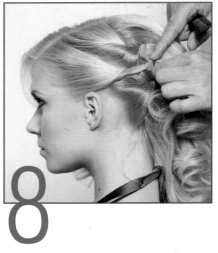

8

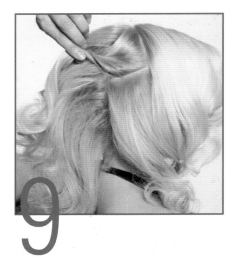

9

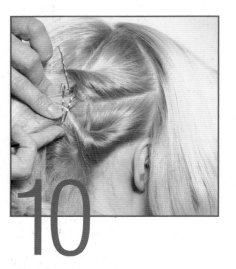

10

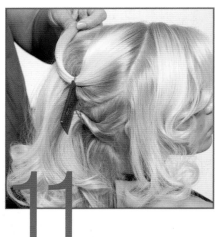

11

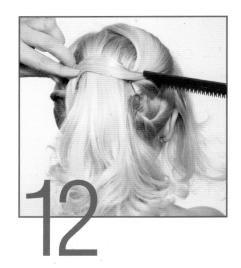

12

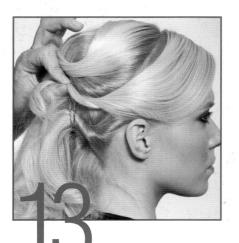

13

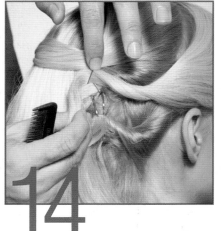

14

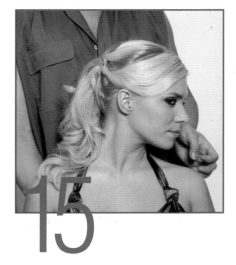

15

7. Gather the hair below this section and twist gently upwards. Secure with hairpins to the spongy base.

8. Gather the remaining hair on this side and twist gently upwards. Secure with a pin to the spongy base, between the two other sections of hair.

9. Move now to the right side of the head, making a diagonal part just above the spongy base. Gather the hair in this section and twist gently upwards, pinning it to the spongy base.

10. Gather the hair below this section and twist it gently upwards. Secure with bobby pins to the spongy base.

11. Divide the remaining hair at the front of the head into front and back sections. Draw the back section towards the spongy base.

12. Using a tail comb for support, draw this hair over the spongy base, towards the left side of the head, and secure with pins.

13. Brush the remaining hair at the front into a wide, flat strip and draw backwards, twisting gently.

14. Secure with a pin to the spongy base between the two other sections of hair.

15. Mist with finishing spray.

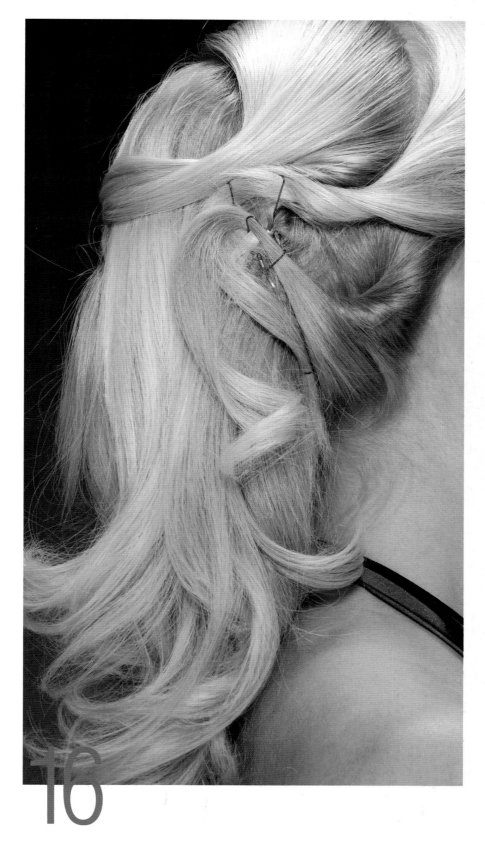

16

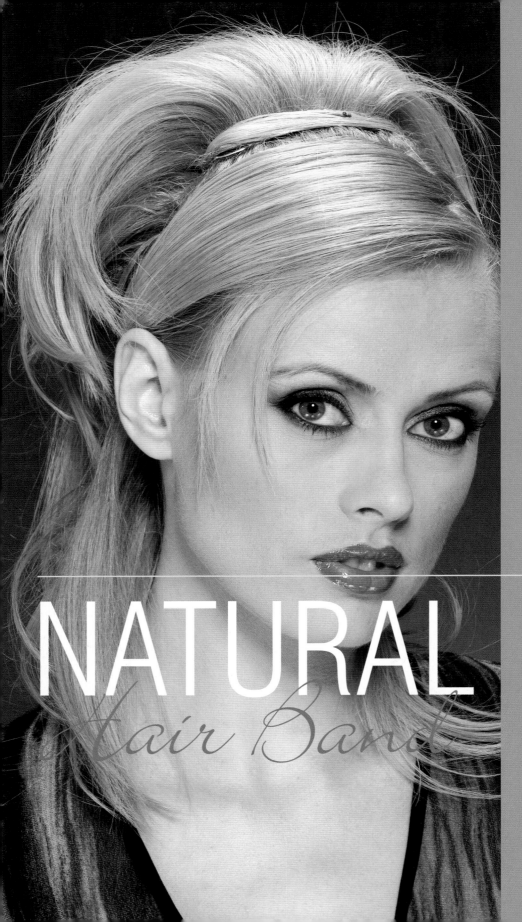

NATURAL
Hair Band

7

Draw the hair backwards and upwards with this refreshing style. It includes a natural hair band, so there is no need to find one that matches your outfit.

1. Wash and blow dry hair upwards. Use a large round brush to add volume.

2. Make a zigzag left side part from the brow to the crown. Gather the hair on either side of the part in clips.

3. Backcomb the hair just behind the crown and mist holding spray at the roots.

4. Blow dry the backcombed hair upwards on medium heat.

5. Move towards the back of the head and backcomb another section of hair. Mist holding spray at the roots.

6. Blow dry the backcombed hair upwards. Continue in this manner until you reach the ear line.

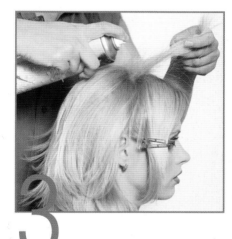

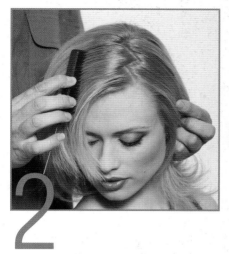

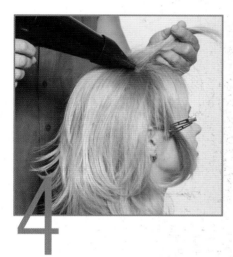

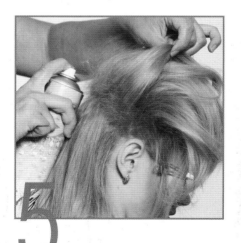

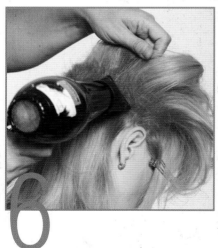

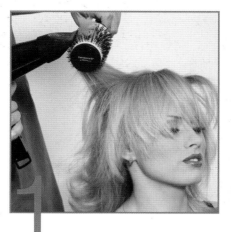

7. Brush the top layer of hair at the crown backwards and secure with a seam of pins at the top.

8. Mist with holding spray and blow dry on medium heat.

9. Move to the hair at the front of the head. Brush the hair on the right side of the part downwards and towards the back.

10. Draw out a lock of hair along the face and pin the rest of the hair at the back.

11. Gather the front hair on the left side of the part and brush backwards and downwards.

12. Secure in place at the back of the head.

13. Draw a lock of hair from behind the pins at the crown. Mist with finishing spray, and brush into a flat strip.

14. Draw the strip over the seam of pins to conceal it. Draw the hair under the seam of pins and secure with a hairpin.

15. Secure the top section of hair at the back of the head with bobby pins.

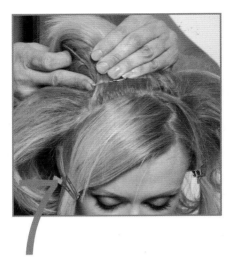

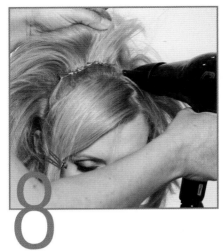

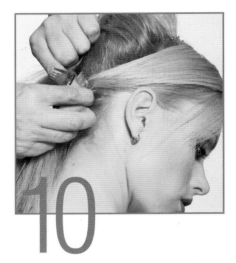

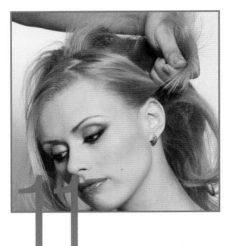

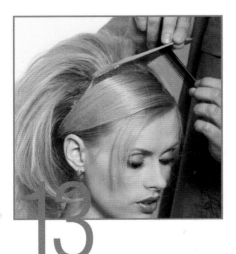

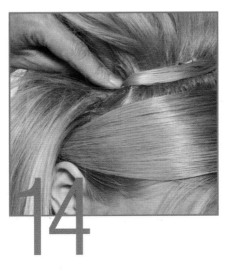

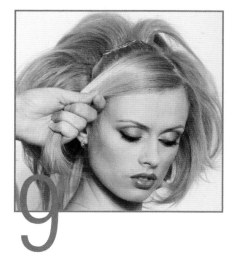

9

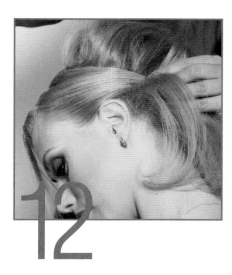

12

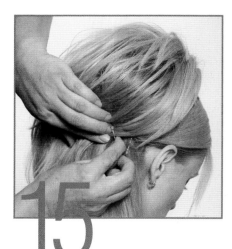

15

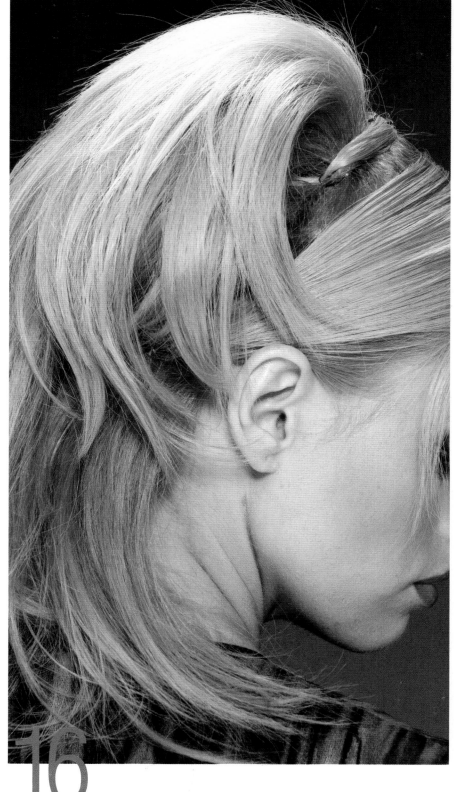

16

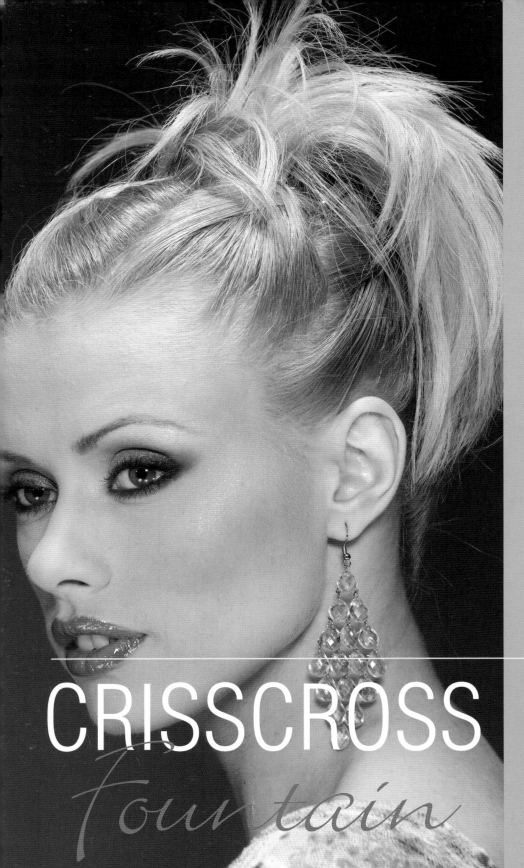

CRISSCROSS
Fountain

8

Cross locks of hair along the sides of the head and gather them at the crown to make a flowing fountain of locks.

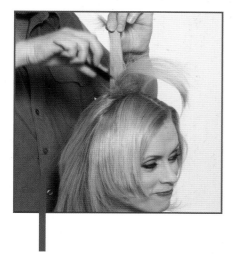

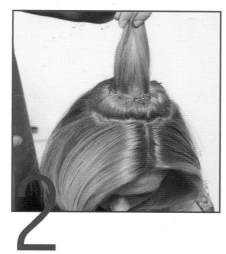

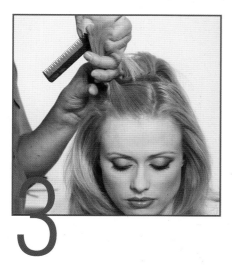

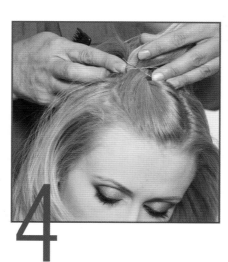

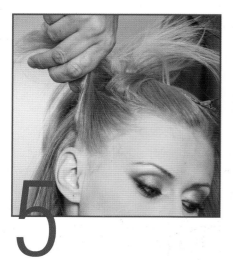

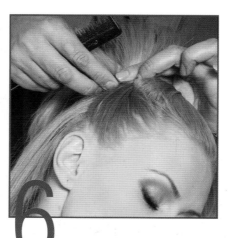

1. Wash and blow dry hair straight. Make a left side part to the crown. Backcomb a circular section of hair at the crown.

2. Brush the backcombed hair upwards and secure with a round seam of pins.

3. Gather hair from a 2-inch section to the right of the part. Brush it upwards while making a half-twist.

4. Secure the hair in place with an X of bobby pins near the seam of pins. Leave the ends loose.

5. Gather hair from a section to the right of the first section and brush the hair upwards while twisting.

6. Secure the hair with bobby pins close to the seam of pins, leaving the ends loose.

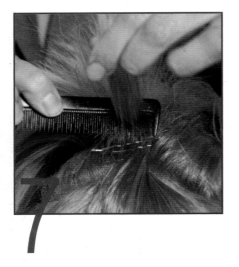

7

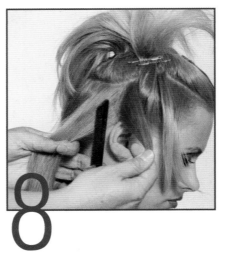

8

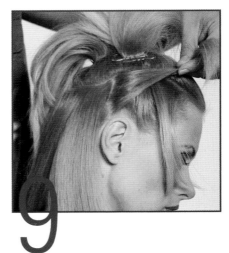

9

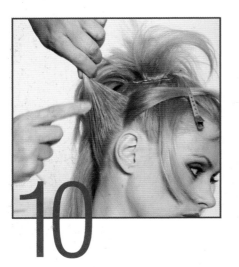

10

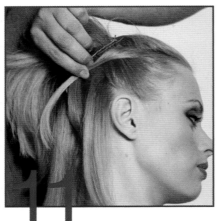

11

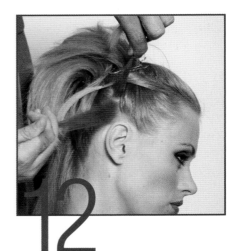

12

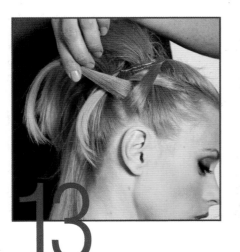

13

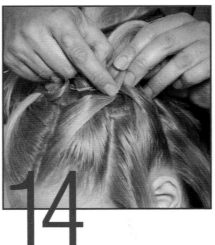

14

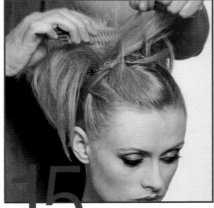

15

7. Backcomb the roots of hair extending from the pins.

8. Divide a section of hair behind the right ear into front and back sections.

9. Brush the front section upwards and forwards. Secure at the front of the head with a clip.

10. Brush the back section of hair upwards and backwards. Make a half-twist in the hair and secure close to the seam of pins, so that the ends of the hair are loose.

11. Release the hair that was clipped in Step 9 and divide into front and back sections. Brush the front section downwards and backwards. Secure in place beside the seam of pins.

12. Divide the back section into top and bottom sections. Draw the bottom section upwards and forwards to make an X of hair and secure near the seam of pins.

13. Draw the top section backwards and secure in place with pins.

14. Repeat on the other side of the head, dividing the hair in sections and making Xs of hair.

15. Backcomb the loose ends of hair and mist with finishing spray.

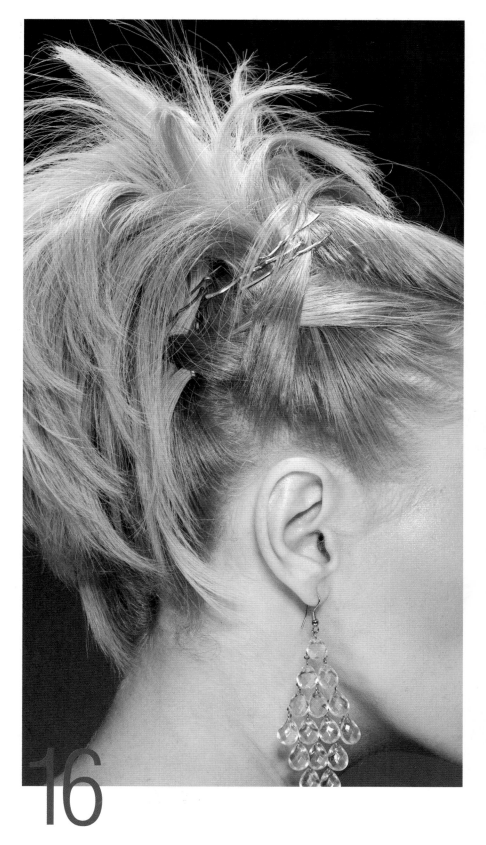

16

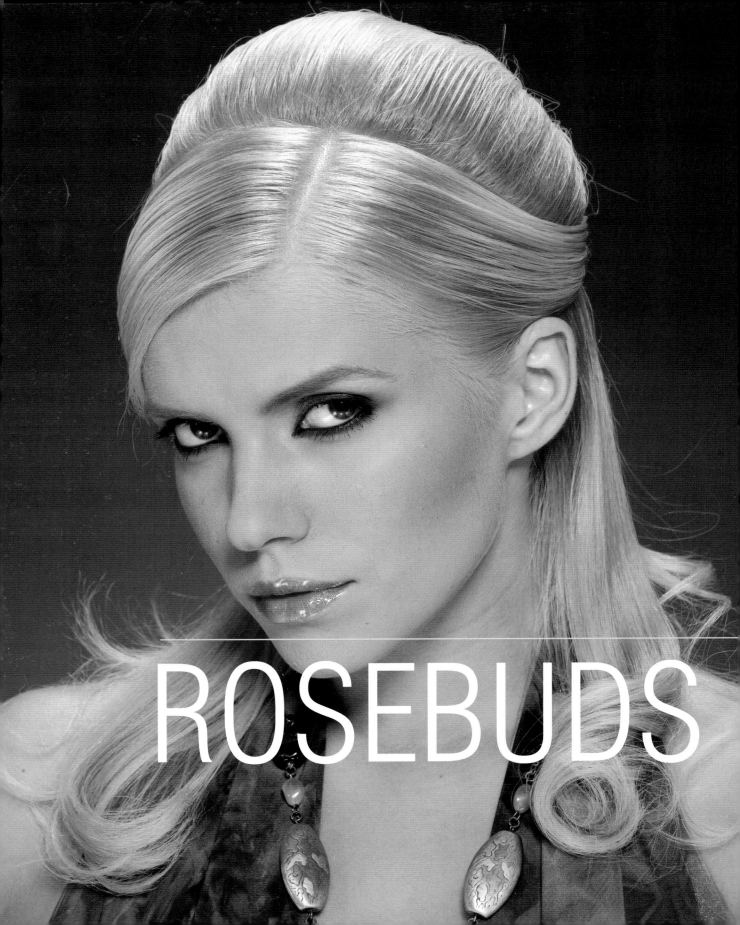

ROSEBUDS

9

The tiny twirls at the back of this style create a flowery effect—no need to add real blossoms to this pretty design.

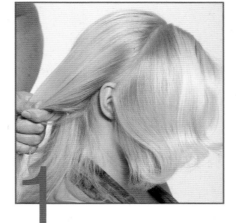

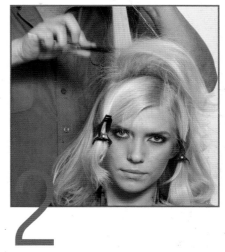

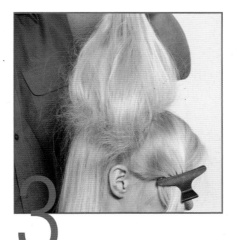

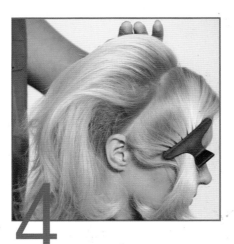

1. Wash and blow dry hair with a diffuser. Divide the hair into front and back sections with a part that extends from ear to ear over the crown.

2. Divide the front section of hair with a left side part, and hold the hair on either side of the part in clips. Backcomb the hair at the crown.

3. Backcomb the hair halfway down the back of the head.

4. Brush the hair just in front of the crown backwards and over the backcombed section.

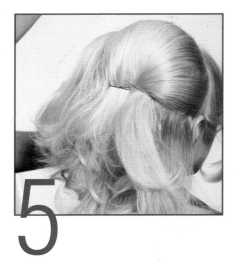

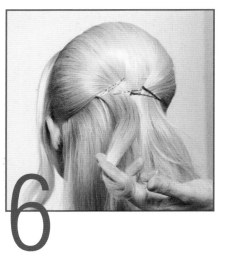

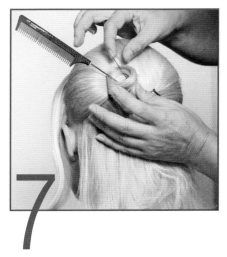

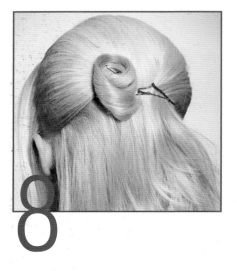

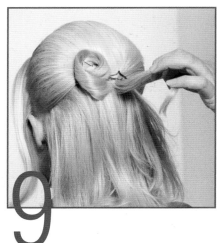

5. Secure the hair with a seam of bobby pins.

6. Draw a lock of hair from the seam of pins.

7. Coil the lock into a flat Figure 6.

8. Use tail combs for support, and secure with hairpins. Mist with holding spray.

9. Make a second Figure 6 beside the first one.

10. Repeat to make a third Figure 6 beside the first two, so that you have three flat Figure 6s at the back of the head hiding the seam of pins.

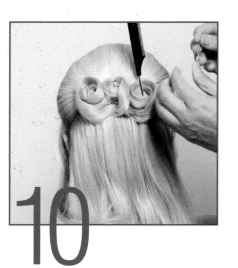

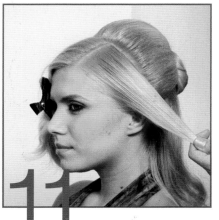

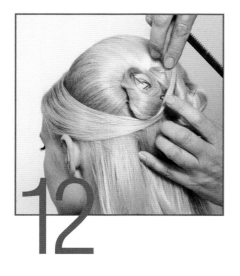

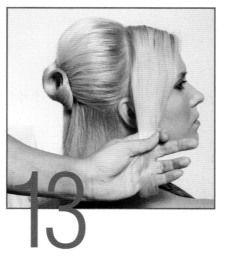

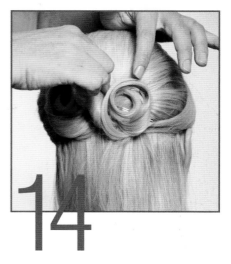

11. Move to the hair at the front of the head. Make a left side part and brush the hair on the left of the part into a flat strip.

12. Draw the hair around the back of the head, looping it around the leftmost Figure 6. Secure with a hairpin.

13. Brush the hair on the right side of the part into a flat strip.

14. Draw the hair around the back of the head, drawing it under the rightmost Figure 6. Secure the hair with a hairpin.

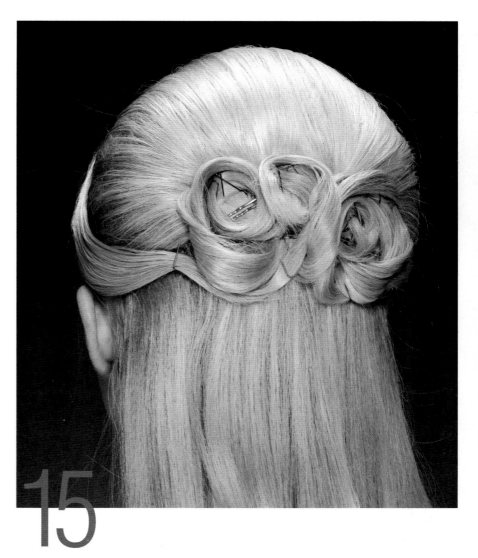

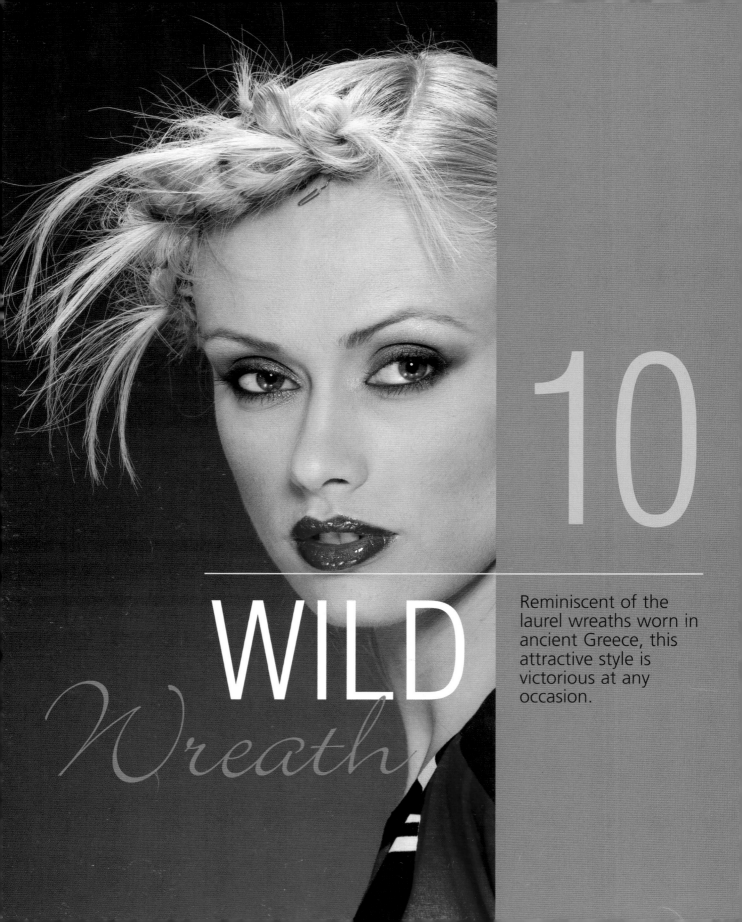

WILD
Wreath

Reminiscent of the laurel wreaths worn in ancient Greece, this attractive style is victorious at any occasion.

1. Wash and blow dry hair straight. Make a triangular part from the brow to the crown that peaks at the crown.

2. Gather the hair in this section in a ponytail at the brow. Mark off a similar section to the right of this section and gather in a ponytail close to the hairline.

3. Continue making ponytails in this manner all along the forehead.

4. Work your way around the right side of the head, across the back of the head, and to the front left side. Leave hair in the last section loose.

5. Move to the first ponytail and coil it into a loose spiral.

6. Push the longest pieces of hair towards the base of the ponytail and secure with a pin. Allow the shorter pieces of hair to extend outwards.

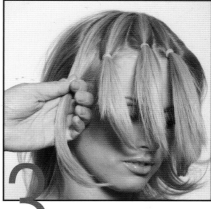

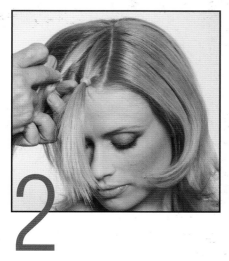
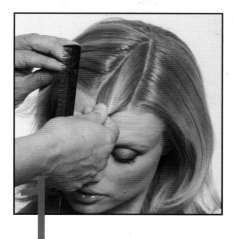
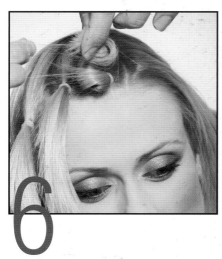
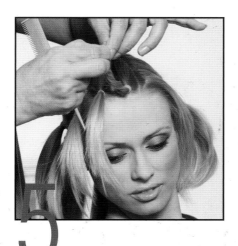
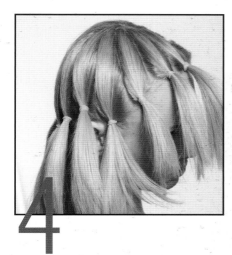

7. Repeat with the next ponytail, twisting it first then coiling it. Secure with a pin, allowing the shorter pieces of hair to extend outwards.

8. Continue coiling the ponytails into loose spirals all along the brow.

9. Move along the back of the head, twisting and coiling the ponytails.

10. Twist and coil the ponytails until you reach the loose section of hair at the front of the head.

11. Brush the hair backwards.

12. Twist the hair inwards and secure with a pin beside the adjacent ponytail, leaving the ends loose.

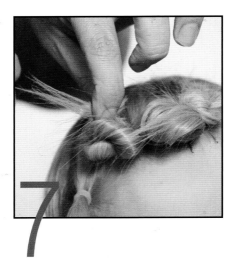

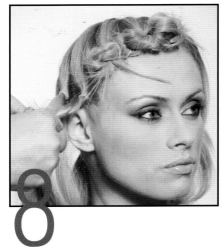

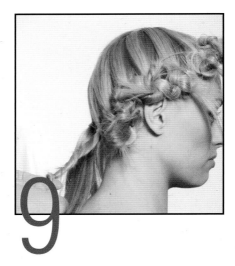

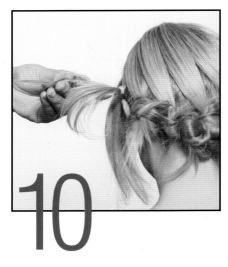

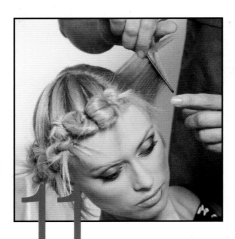

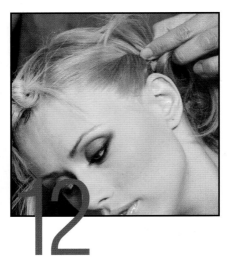

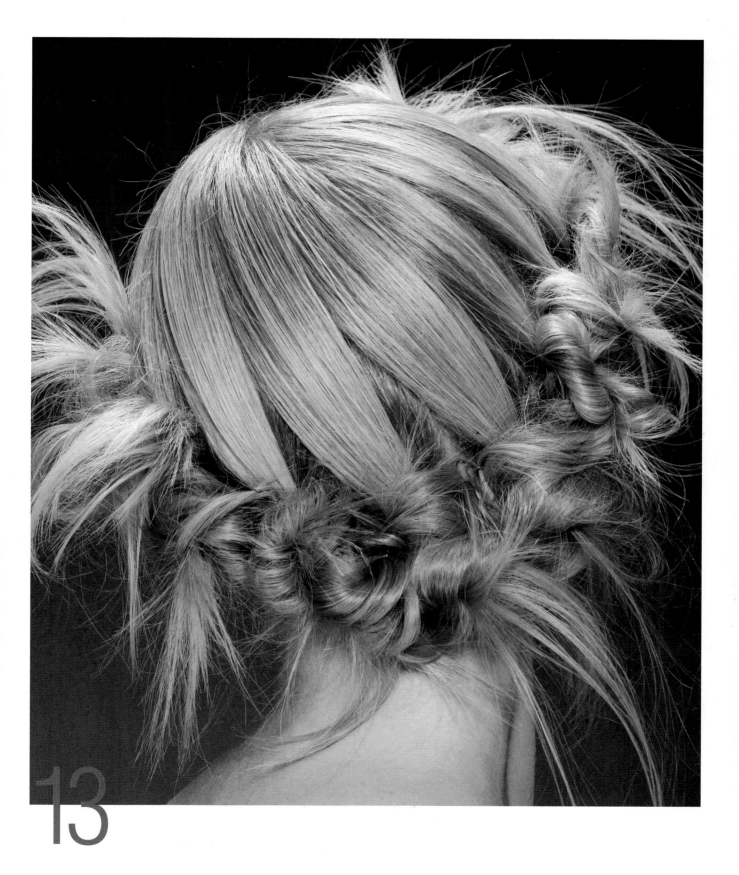

13

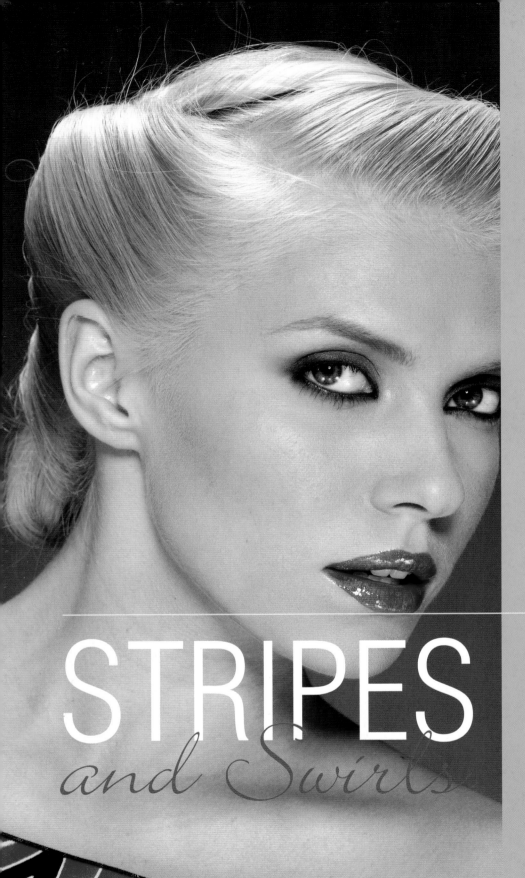

STRIPES
and Swirls

Combine diagonal stripes along the back of the head with elegant coils at the nape of the neck.

1. Wash and blow dry hair straight. Divide the hair into front and back sections with a part that extends from ear to ear over the crown. Divide the back section into three vertical sections.

2. Gather the hair in the middle section in a clip at the top of the head. Backcomb the hair in the left and right sections to make two spongy bases.

3. Make a horizontal part 1 inch above the neck in the middle section and brush the hair downwards. Make a diagonal part just above this section on the right side. Mist the hair with holding spray and twist tightly at the roots. Pin the twisted hair to the spongy base on the left side.

4. Make a diagonal part above this section and brush the hair towards the right side of the head. Mist with holding spray.

5. Twist the hair tightly at the roots while drawing it to the spongy base on the right side.

6. Secure the twisted hair on the right side of the head.

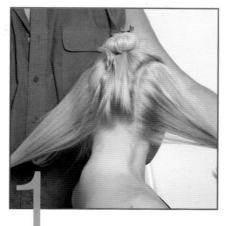
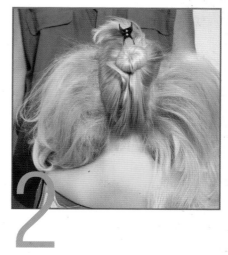

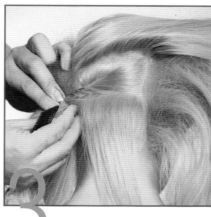

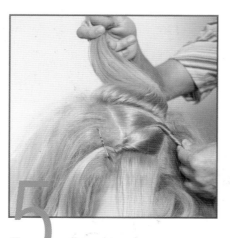

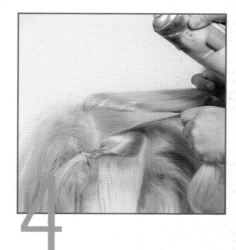
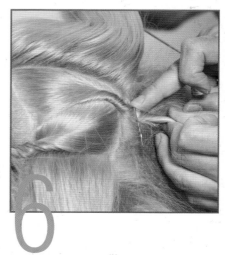

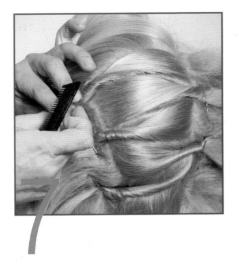

7

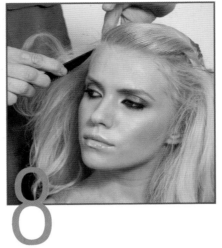

8

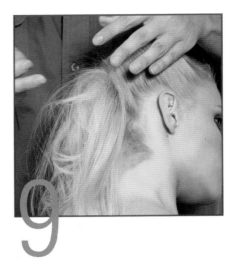

9

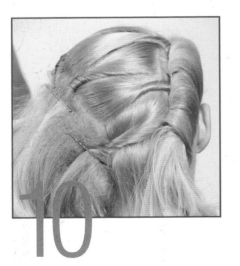

10

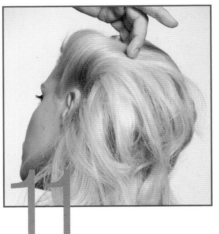

11

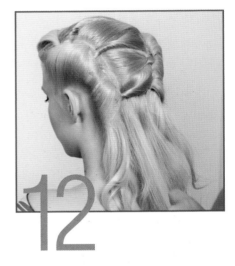

12

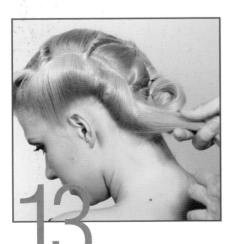

13

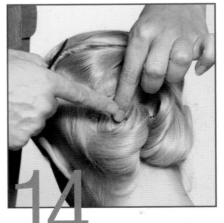

14

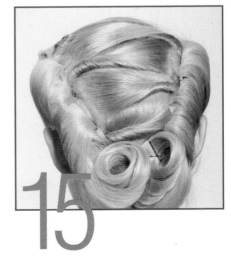

15

7. Continue in this manner, working your way upwards and alternating direction each time.

8. Brush back the bangs and twist, drawing the hair from the right side of the brow and pinning it to the spongy base on the left side.

9. Brush the loose hair on the right side of the head upwards.

10. Tuck the loose hair over the pins securing the twisted hair, and secure with hairpins.

11. Repeat on the left side of the head.

12. In this manner, make two thick rolls of hair on either side of the head. These rolls should conceal the pins securing the twisted hair.

13. Divide the loose hair at the back of the head into two sections. Coil the hair on the right side upwards into a soft flat Figure 6 and secure with hairpins at the nape of the neck. Mist hair with holding spray to hold.

14. Repeat with the hair on the left side, coiling the hair into a soft flat Figure 6.

15. Mist with finishing spray.

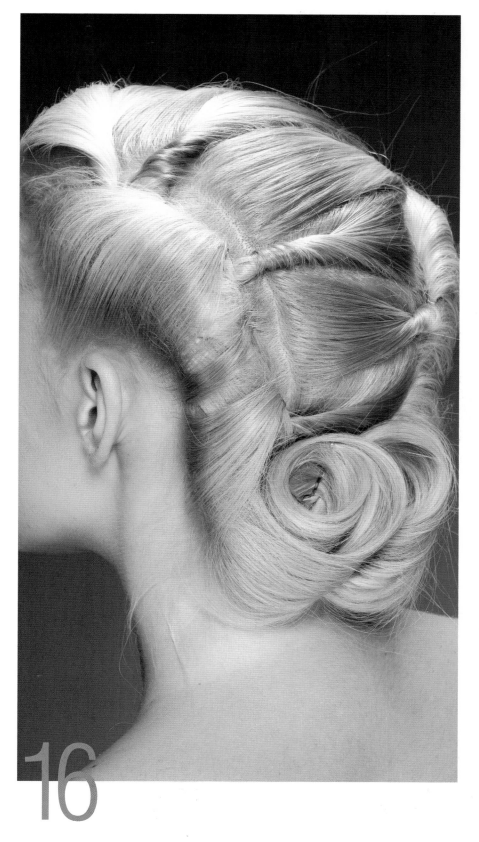

16

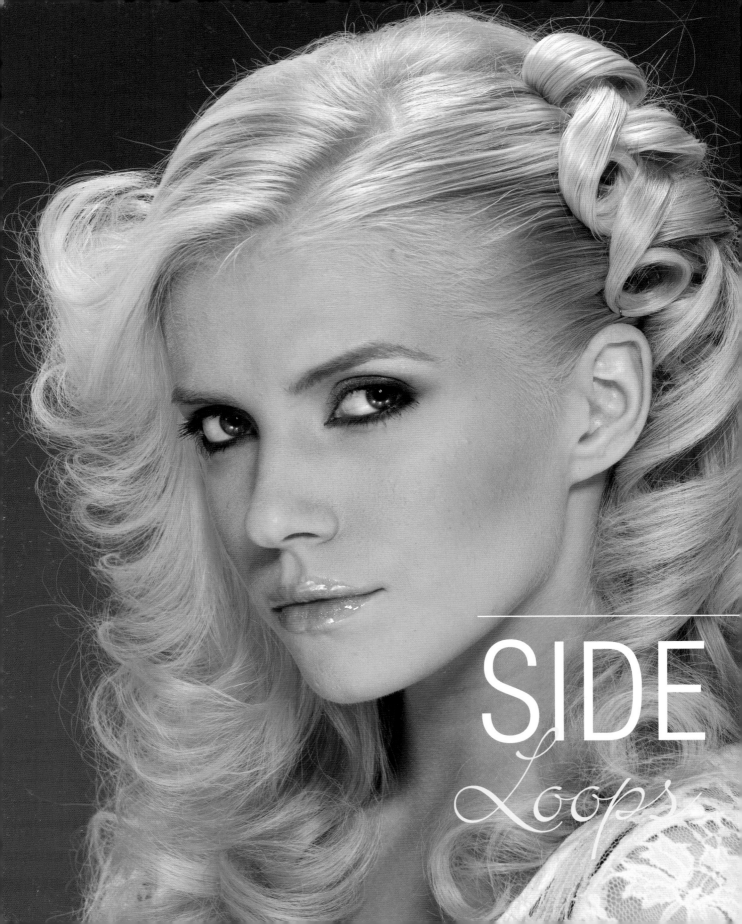

SIDE *Loops*

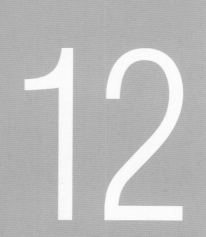

This asymmetrical design is flirtatious and fun. Lovely style for an afternoon affair that calls for a loose, almost casual look.

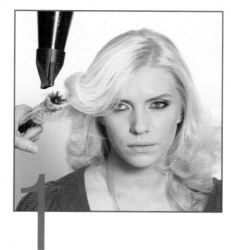

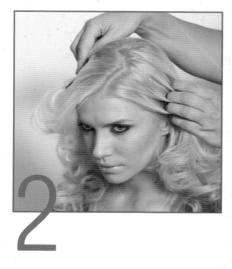

1. Wash and blow dry curly. Use a round brush to add volume.

2. Make a zigzag left side part.

3. Make a part from the crown to the back of the left ear. Hold the front hair in a clip and back-comb the hair behind the part.

4. Backcomb the hair in an arc towards the ear to make a spongy arc base behind the ear.

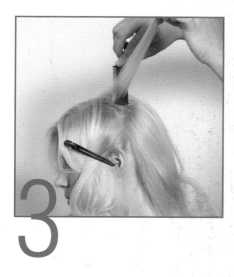

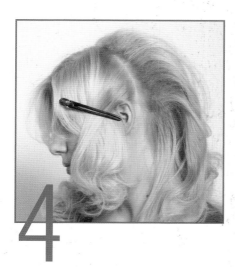

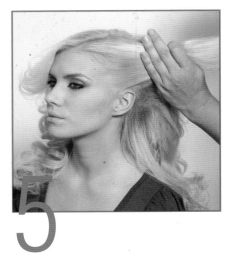

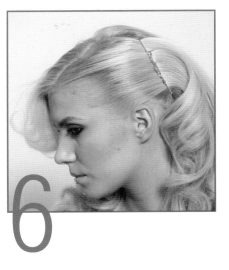

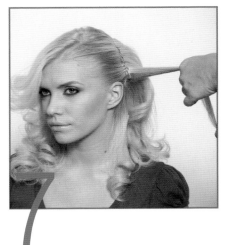

5. Brush the front hair backwards and over the spongy base.

6. Secure the hair with a seam of pins behind the left ear.

7. Draw a lock of hair from behind the seam of pins. Mist with holding spray and brush into a flat strip.

8. Using a tail comb for support, roll the hair over a finger to form a loop and secure with a bobby pin, leaving the ends loose.

9. Draw another lock of hair, mist with holding spray, and brush into a flat strip.

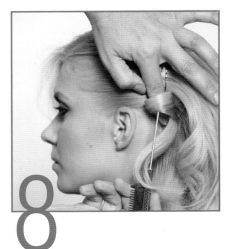

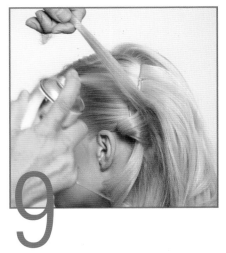

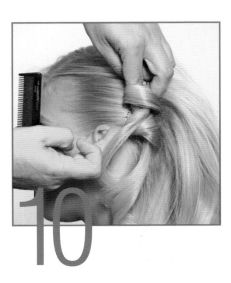

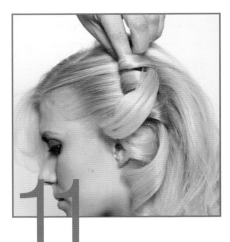

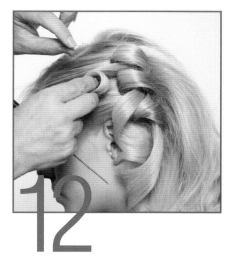

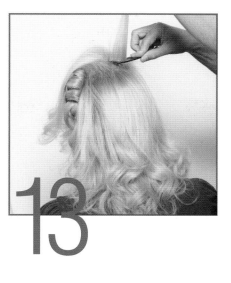

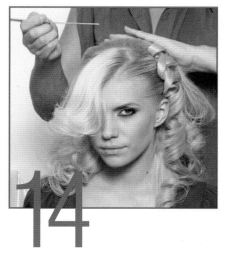

10. Roll the lock in a similar manner to form another loop. Secure with a bobby pin, leaving the ends loose.

11. Draw another lock of hair, just above the first two locks, and roll it into a third loop, leaving the ends loose.

12. Coil the ends into a flat Figure 6.

13. Backcomb the hair at the crown.

14. Brush some of the front hair over the backcombed hair, leaving the rest of the hair loose.

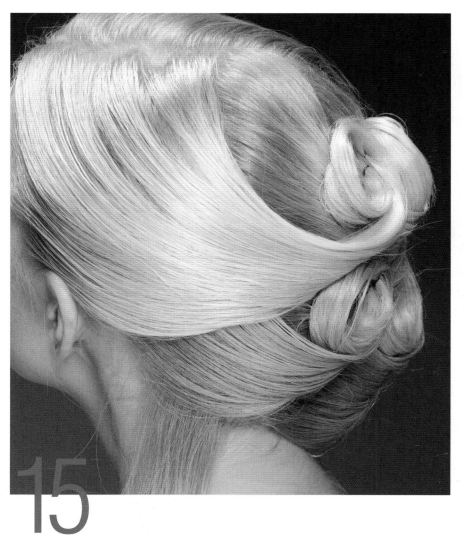

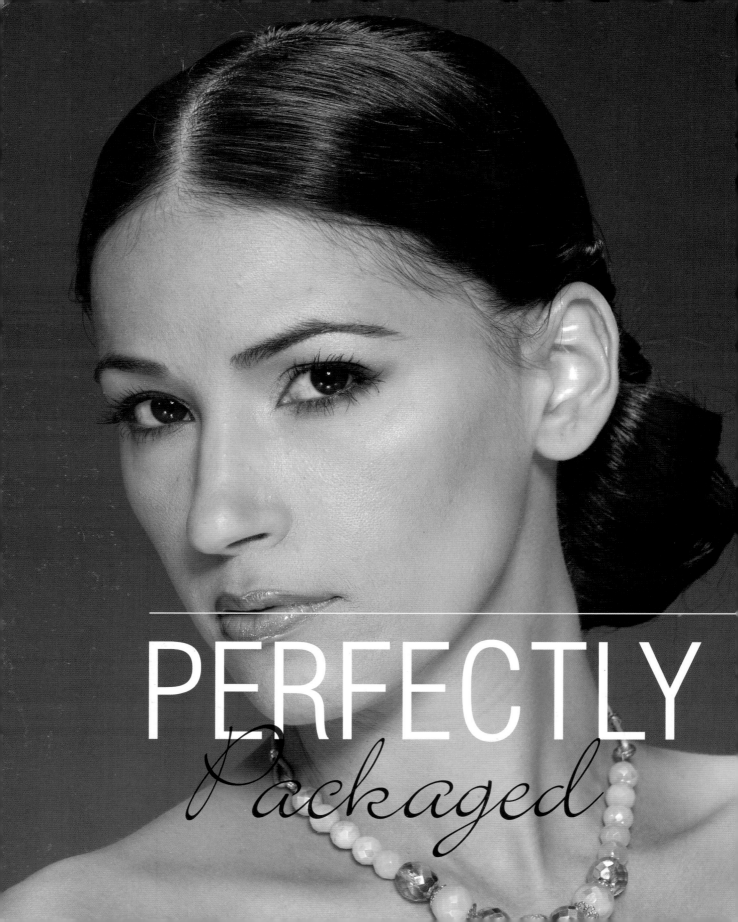

PERFECTLY
Packaged

13

1. Wash and blow dry hair straight. Divide the hair into front and back sections with a part that extends from ear to ear over the crown. Make a center part in the front hair and gather the hair on either side of the part in clips. Make a low ponytail with the back hair. Draw a lock of hair from the ponytail, mist with holding spray, and brush into a flat strip. Wrap the strip around the base of the ponytail to conceal the elastic band.

2. Place another elastic band a few inches below the first one to make a closed ponytail.

3. Divide the hair after the second elastic band into two sections.

4. Fold the hair inwards so that the second elastic band is under the first elastic band.

Wrap your hair like a present for a very special party. With an almost Victorian elegance, this style has unmistakable class.

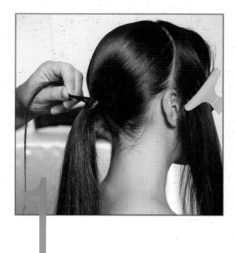

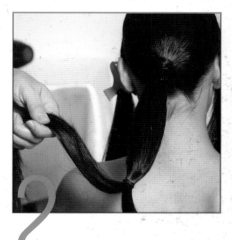

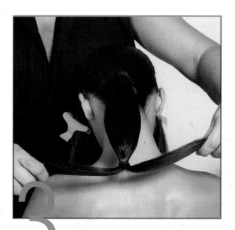

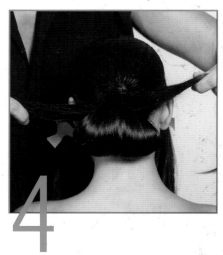

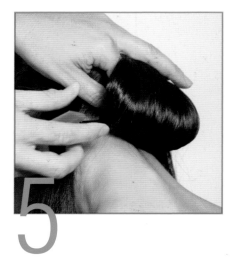

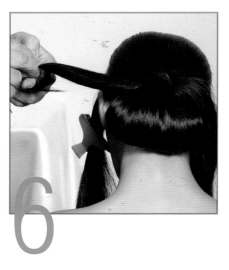

5. Secure the folded hair to the head with bobby pins on either side to make an upside-down fan.

6. Brush the hair extending from the left side of the fan into a flat strip. Roll the hair downwards over a finger into a loop.

7. Secure the loop under the upside-down fan with a bobby pin.

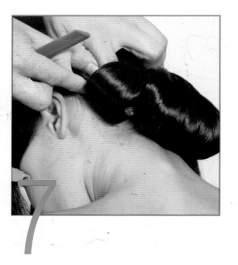

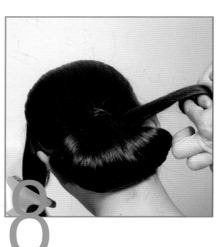

8. Make a loop with the hair on the left side of the fan in a similar manner.

9. Secure with a bobby pin under the upside-down fan.

10. Move to the front section and brush out the hair on the right side of the part.

11. Twist the hair tightly upwards.

12. Draw the twist backwards and secure with a pin just above the upside-down fan.

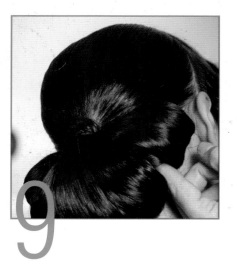

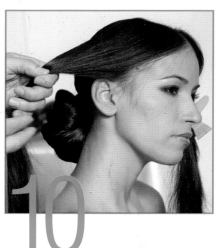

13. Make sure the hair stays twisted as you coil it around a finger to make a twisted spiral.

14. Secure the spiral to the right side of the upside-down fan with a hairpin.

15. Repeat on the other side of the head, making another twisted spiral on the left side of the head. Secure with a hairpin just above the upside-down fan.

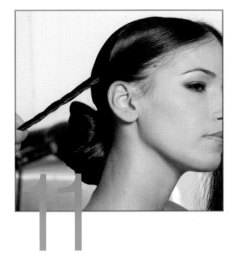

11

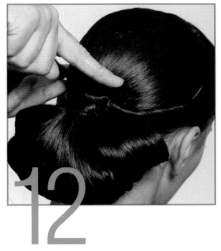

12

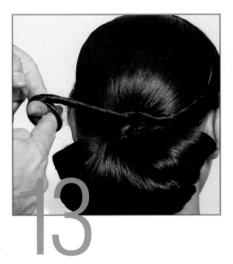

13

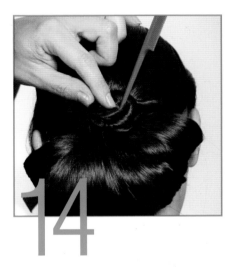

14

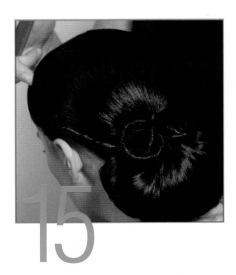

15

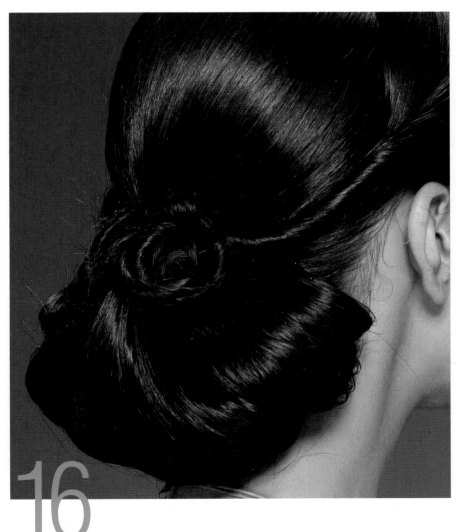

16

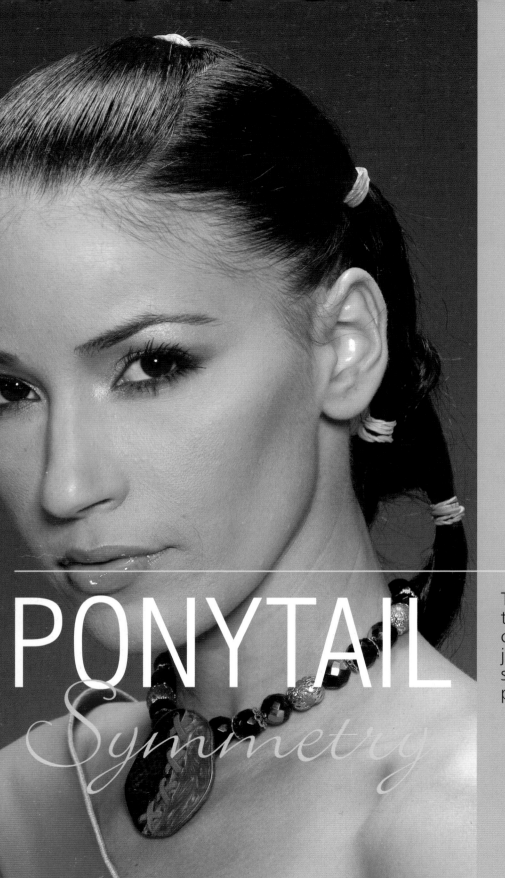

14

PONYTAIL
Symmetry

Tidy and distinct, this style features a collection of ponytails joined together in a seemingly intricate pattern.

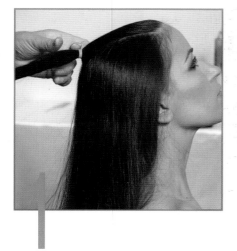

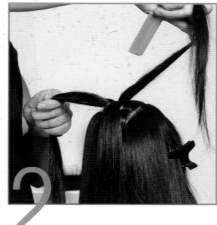

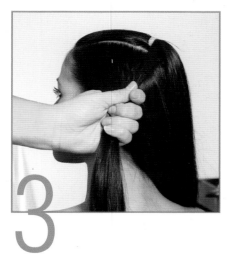

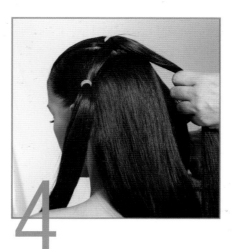

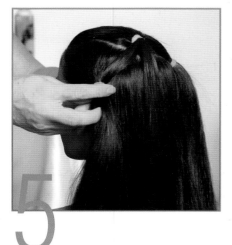

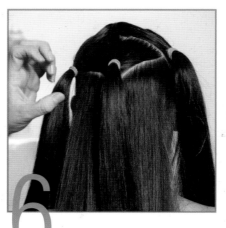

1. Wash and blow dry hair straight. Make a triangular part that includes all of the bangs and peaks at the crown. Gather the hair in this section in a ponytail that is close to the roots.

2. Divide the ponytail into three sections.

3. Join the leftmost section of the ponytail with the hair to the left of the ponytail to make a ponytail that is between the left ear and the first ponytail.

4. Repeat on other side of the head, making a ponytail that joins the rightmost section of hair in the top ponytail with the loose hair to the right of the ponytail.

5. The middle section of the top ponytail should be loose.

6. Make a triangular part that extends from the right ponytail to the left ponytail and peaks in the middle of the head. Gather the loose hair from the middle section of the top ponytail and the hair from this triangular section into a fourth ponytail that is directly below the top ponytail.

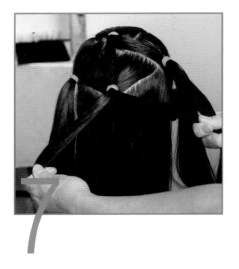

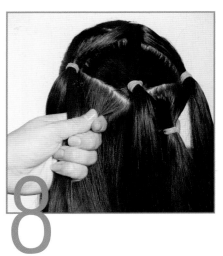

7. Divide this ponytail into two sections.

8. Gather half of the hair in the ponytail on the left with hair from a triangular section on the left side of the head. Join with the hair in the left section of the center ponytail and form another ponytail. Repeat on the other side of the head.

9. There should be six ponytails. Divide the two ponytails on the bottom into two sections.

10. Gather the sections closest to each other, and the loose hair between them, into a ponytail at the nape of the neck. There should now be seven ponytails; five of these ponytails have loose ends.

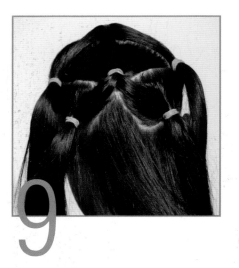

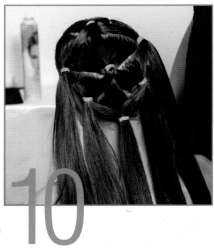

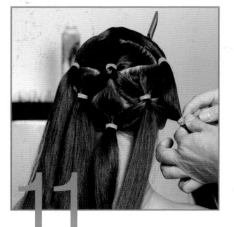

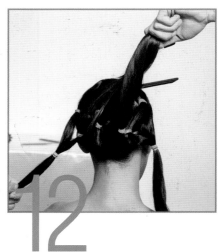

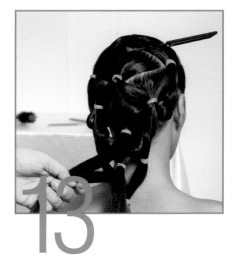

11. Gather the hair from the rightmost ponytail, and half of the hair from the adjacent ponytail, and make a ponytail.

12. Repeat on the other side of the head, joining the hair from the leftmost ponytail with half of the hair from the adjacent ponytail. Raise all of the hair except for the rightmost and leftmost ponytails. Draw these two ponytails together under the lifted hair and join in a ponytail.

13. Lower the hair. Join half of the hair in the middle ponytail and half of the hair in the bottom ponytail into a ponytail that is under the hair that was lifted.

14. Join the other halves of these two ponytails in another ponytail. This ponytail should be above the hair that was lifted previously.

15. Join these two ponytails in a single ponytail.

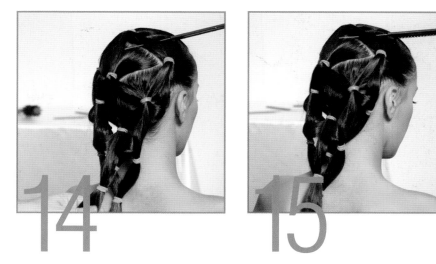

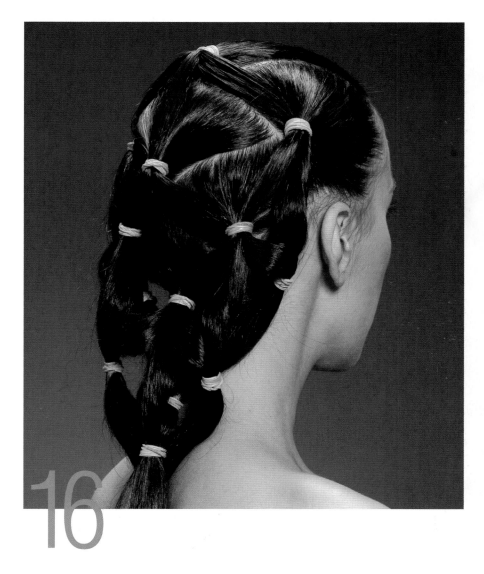

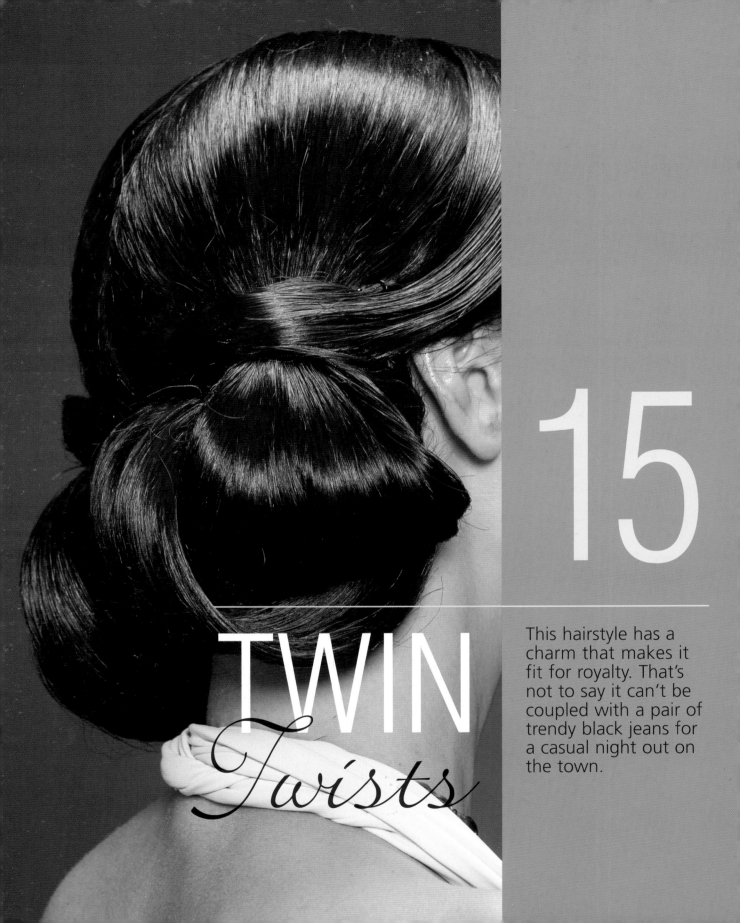

15

TWIN
Twists

This hairstyle has a charm that makes it fit for royalty. That's not to say it can't be coupled with a pair of trendy black jeans for a casual night out on the town.

1. Wash and blow dry hair straight. Divide the hair into front and back sections with a part that extends from ear to ear over the crown. Divide the back section with a center part, and make low ponytails behind each ear.

2. Brush the hair in the right ponytail into a wide strip.

3. Mist with holding spray and blow dry.

4. Fold the strip inwards to make an upside-down fan and secure with a pin near the base of the ponytail. Leave the hair that extends beyond the fan loose.

5. Wrap the loose hair under the fan and draw it upwards so that it covers the elastic band. Secure in place with a pin.

6. Repeat on the other side of the head, folding the hair in the ponytail to make an upside-down fan.

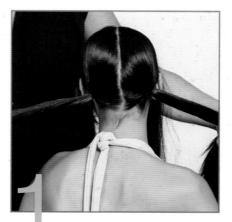

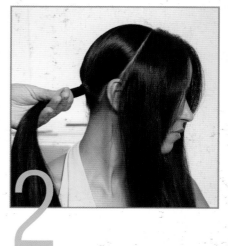

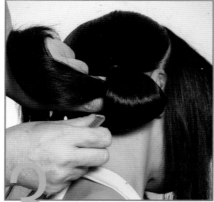

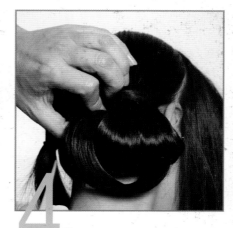

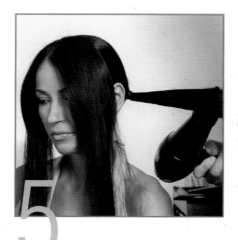

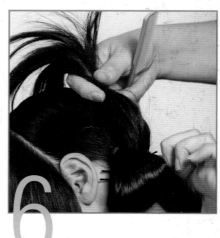

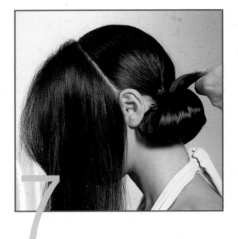

7

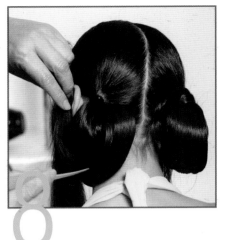

8

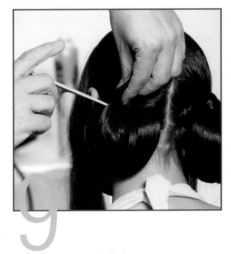

9

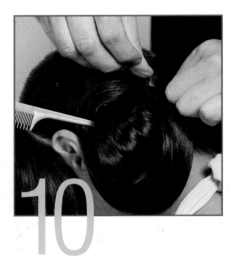

10

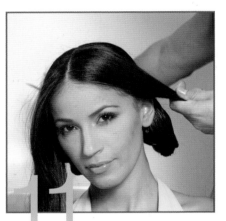

11

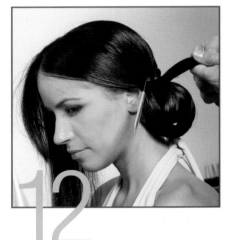

12

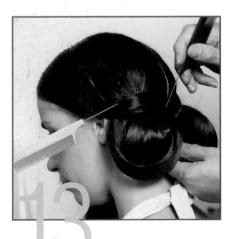

13

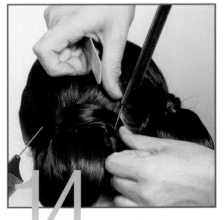

14

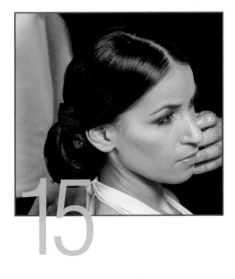

15

7. Leave the hair that extends beyond the fan loose.

8. Wrap the loose hair under the fan.

9. Draw it upwards around the front of the fan.

10. Secure near the base of the ponytail so that it covers the elastic band.

11. Brush the front hair on the left side backwards.

12. Hold the hair in place with a tail comb, and mist with finishing spray.

13. Wrap the hair over the top of the fan and towards the back of the head.

14. Secure with a bobby pin.

15. Repeat on the other side of the head.

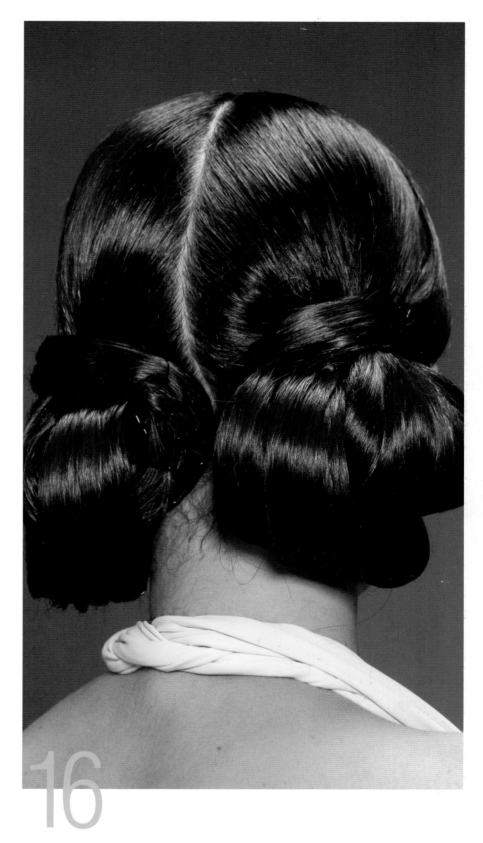

16

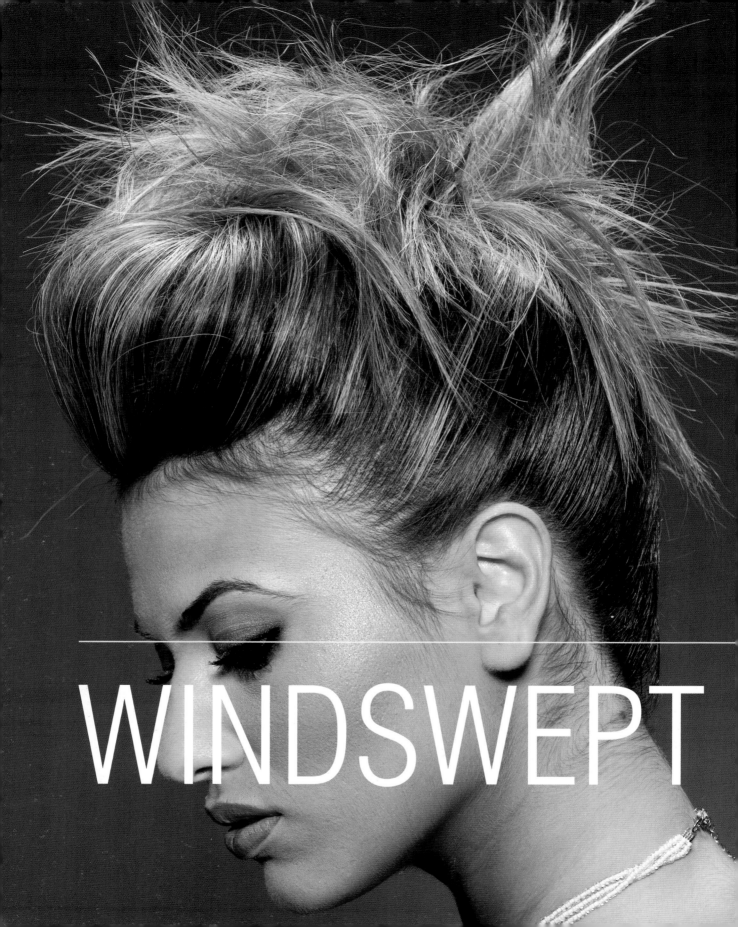

WINDSWEPT

16

1. Wash and blow dry hair. Backcomb the hair starting at the crown.

2. Work your way down the head, densely backcombing all of the hair.

3. Bend over and brush the hair at the back of the head upwards, from the nape of the neck and until the ears.

4. Secure the back hair at the top of the head with a seam of pins.

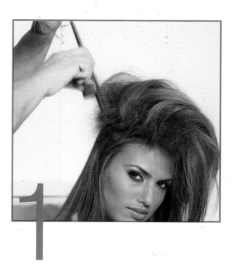

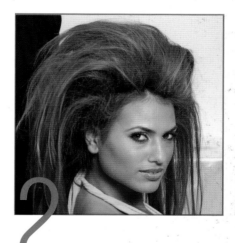

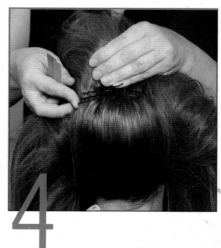

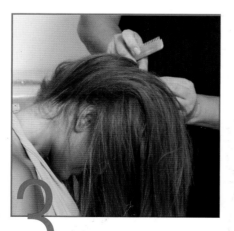

Gather long hair at the top of the head in this lively style. It features a smooth front and untamed ends for a look that is arrestingly surprising.

5. Brush the hair to the left side of the head upwards and backwards.

6. Twist the hair into an inwards roll, leaving the ends loose and upwards. Secure with hairpins just over the seam of bobby pins.

7. Brush the hair on the right side upwards and backwards.

8. Make another inwards roll, leaving the ends loose and upwards.

9. Secure with pins at the crown so that the two rolls form a triangle at the back of the head.

10. Brush the hair at the front of the head upwards.

11. Draw the front hair backwards so that it covers the top of the triangle.

12. Twist the hair towards the back to make a closed U shape and secure with hairpins at the top of the triangle, leaving the ends loose.

13. Brush the front hair upwards and mist with holding spray.

14. Backcomb the loose ends at the top of the head, orienting them in every direction.

15. Mist with finishing spray.

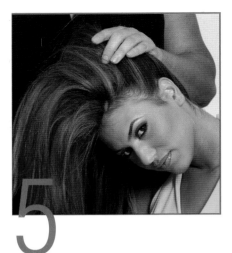

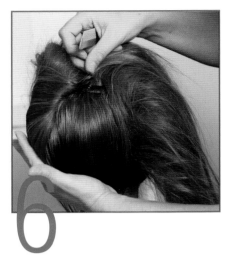

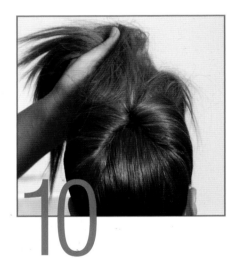

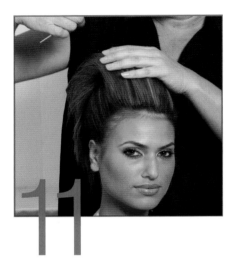

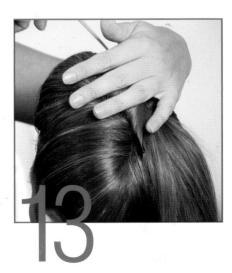

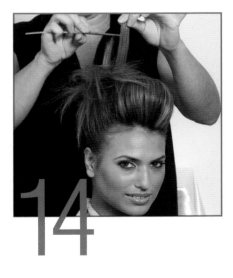

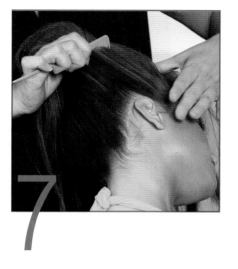

7

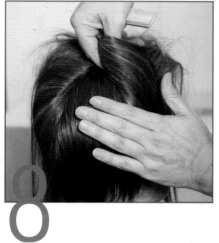

8

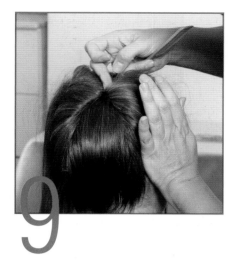

9

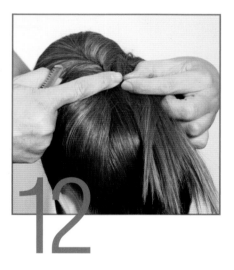

12

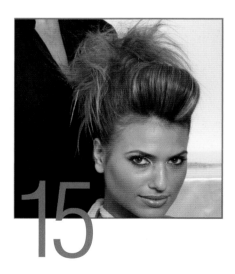

15

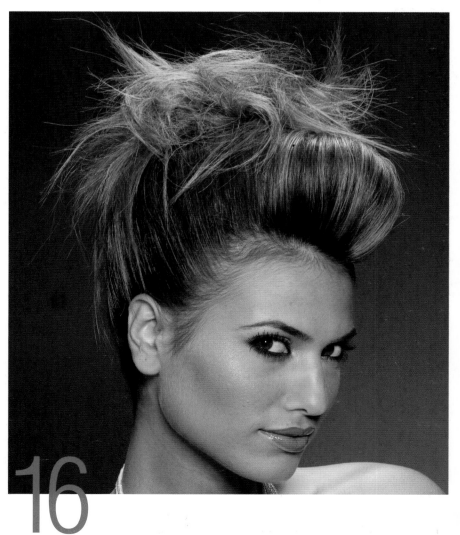

16

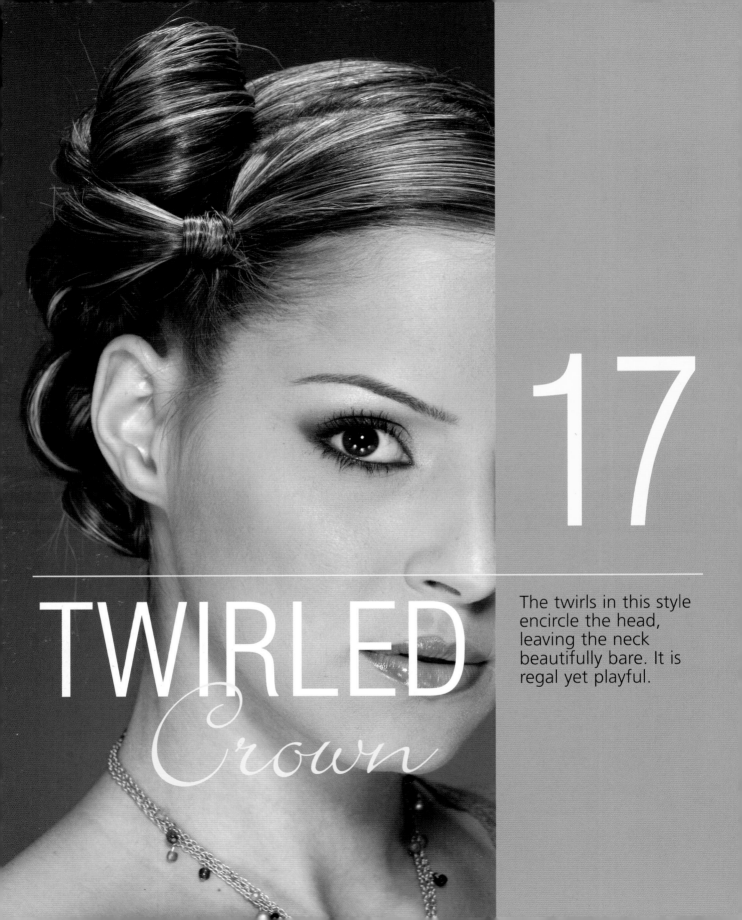

17

TWIRLED *Crown*

The twirls in this style encircle the head, leaving the neck beautifully bare. It is regal yet playful.

1. Wash and blow dry hair straight. Make a diagonal part from the left eyebrow to the top of the right ear.

2. Gather the hair in this section in a ponytail just above the right ear.

3. Make a part over the top of the head and gather the hair in a similar ponytail above the left ear.

4. Make a diagonal part that extends from the ponytail on the left side to the middle of the right ear. Gather the hair in this section in a ponytail that is below the first ponytail.

5. Repeat on the other side, making a diagonal part from the second ponytail on the right and to the left side of the neck. Collect the hair in a ponytail under the first ponytail on the left side.

6. Continue in this manner, making diagonal parts and ponytails on either side of the head.

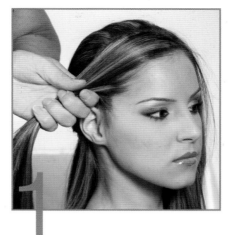

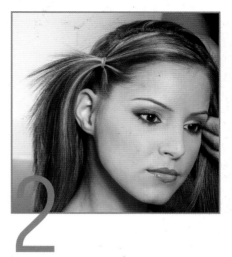

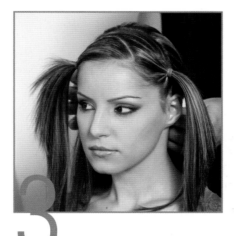

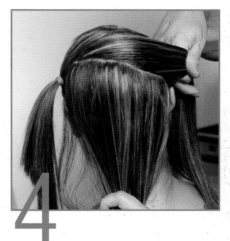

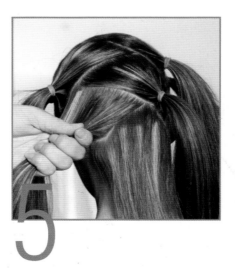

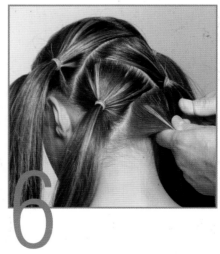

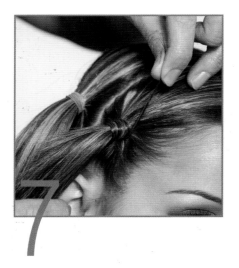

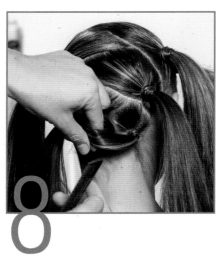

7. Draw a lock of hair from the top ponytail, mist with holding spray, and brush into a flat strip. Wrap the strip around the base of the ponytail to conceal the elastic band. Repeat with the other ponytails to conceal all of the elastic bands.

8. Start with the ponytail at the bottom, and wrap it upwards and inwards around a finger.

9. Use a tail comb for support and wrap the hair into a standing Figure 6. Secure with a hairpin.

10. Move to the next ponytail at the bottom, and divide the hair into two sections.

11. Wrap the bottommost section around a finger to form a standing Figure 6 facing the first Figure 6. Secure with a hairpin.

12. Wrap the other section upwards around a finger to form a standing Figure 6 and secure with a hairpin.

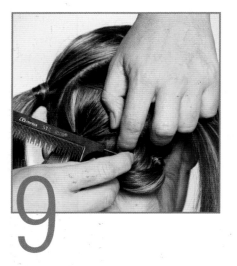

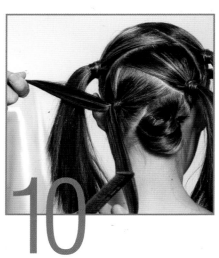

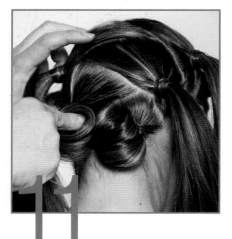

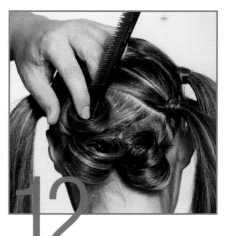

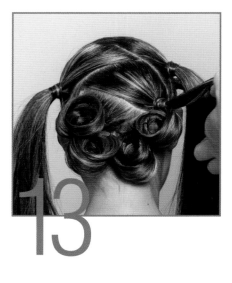

13. Repeat with the other ponytails, dividing each ponytail into two sections and making standing Figure 6s in each section.

14. Work your way from the bottom of the head towards the top.

15. Draw the top ponytails backwards. Wrap into standing Figure 6s, and secure with hairpins.

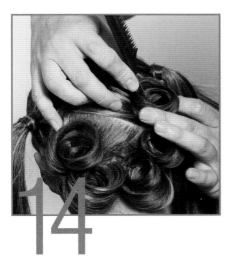

14

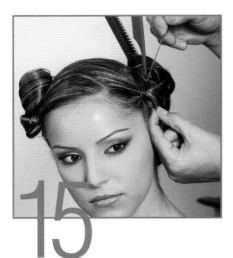

15

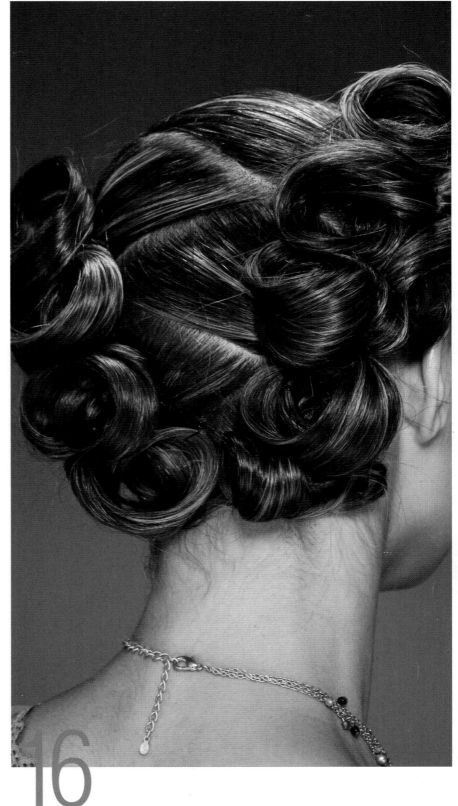

16

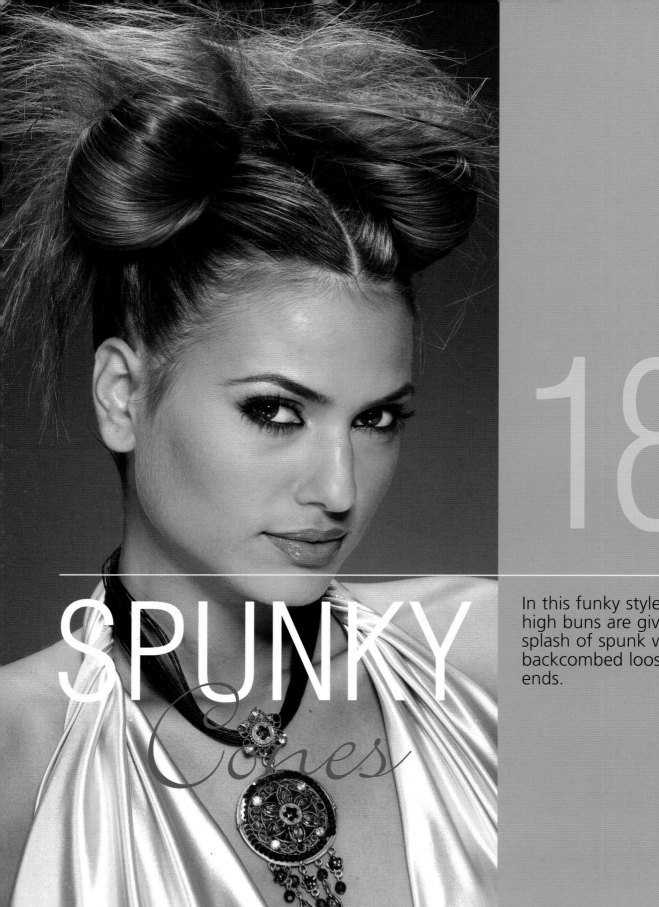

18

SPUNKY
Cones

In this funky style, two high buns are given a splash of spunk with backcombed loose ends.

1. Wash and blow dry hair straight. Divide hair with a middle part and make high ponytails on either side of the part. Draw a lock of hair from each ponytail, mist with holding spray, and brush into flat strips. Wrap the strips around the base of each ponytail to conceal the elastic bands.

2. Lightly backcomb the ponytail on the right.

3. Brush the hair into a flat strip. Mist with holding spray and blow dry.

4. Twist the strip of hair outwards and forwards.

5. Draw the hair upwards, using tail combs for support.

6. Now draw the hair towards the back of the head, to make a cone.

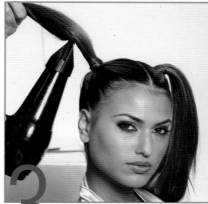
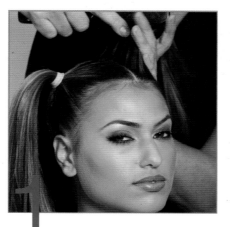
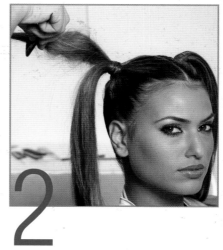
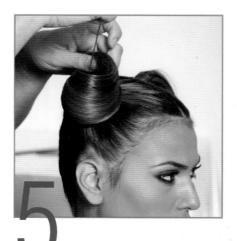
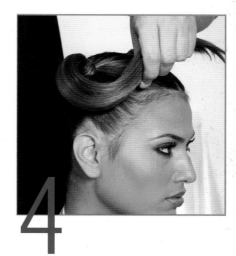

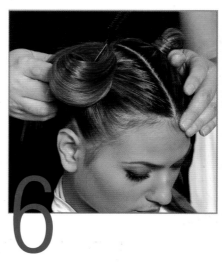

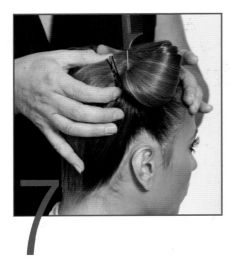

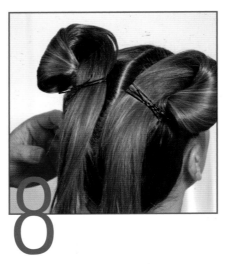

7. Secure the hair with bobby pins at the back of the head, leaving the ends loose and downwards.

8. Repeat with the left ponytail, backcombing the hair, brushing it into a flat strip, then twisting it outwards and towards the front of the head. Form a cone that is a mirror image of the first one and secure with bobby pins at the back of the head, leaving the ends loose and downwards.

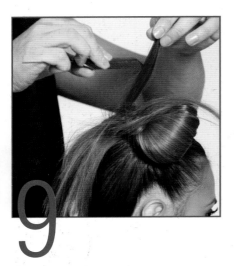

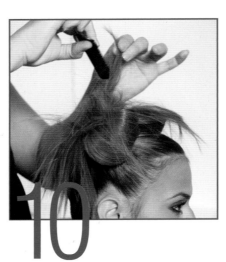

9. Lightly backcomb the loose ends at the back of the head.

10. Orient some of the back-combed hair so that it conceals the pins.

11. Orient the remaining back-combed hair to create a high tangle.

12. The final style is a striking combination of smooth cones and tangled ends.

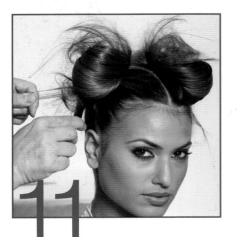

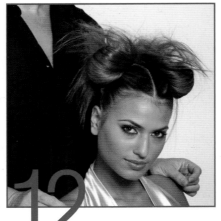

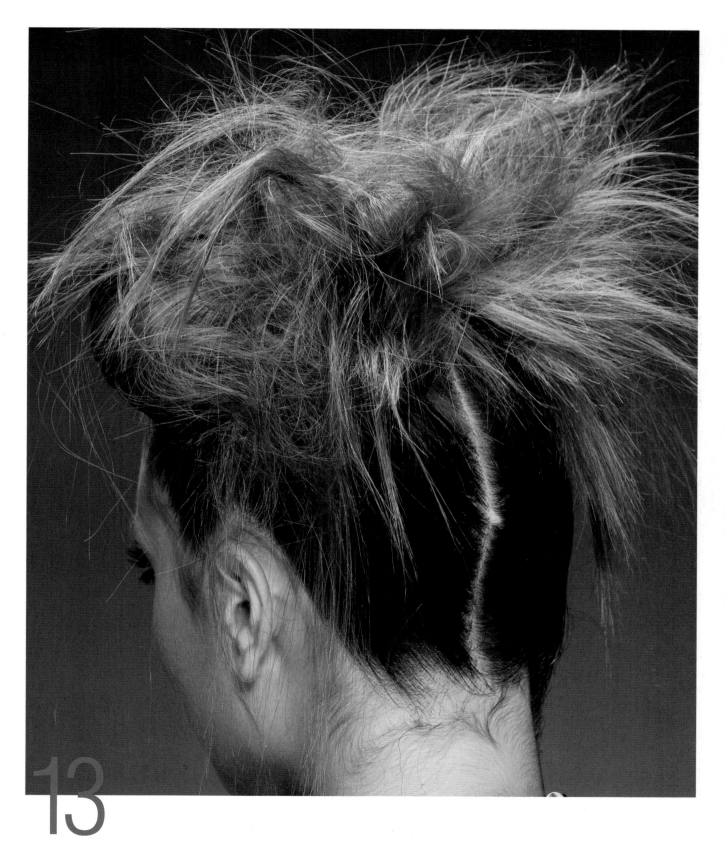

13

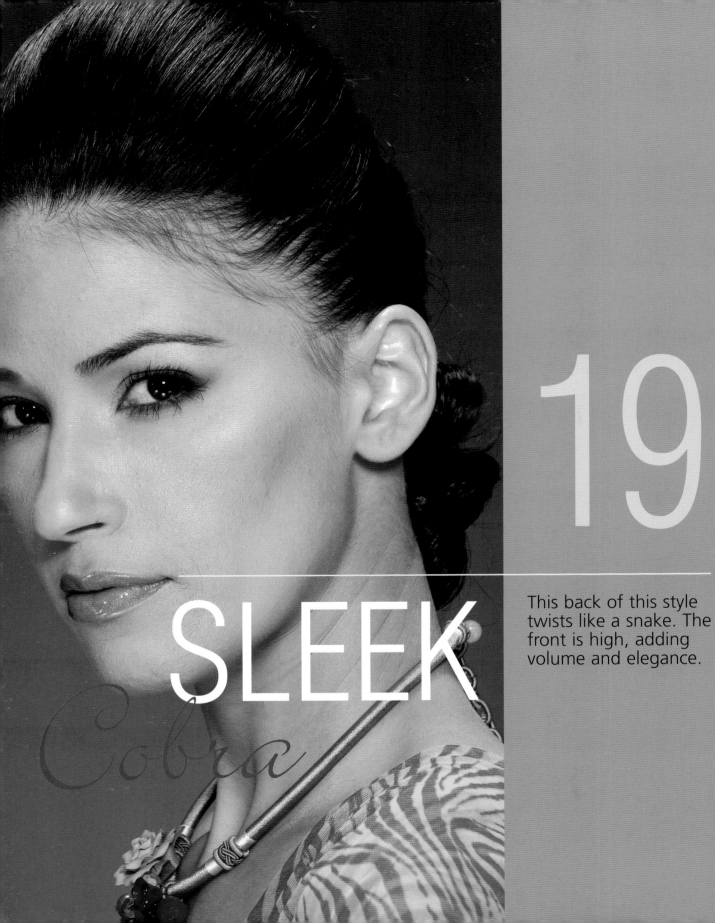

19

SLEEK

Cobra

This back of this style
twists like a snake. The
front is high, adding
volume and elegance.

1. Wash and blow dry hair straight. Gather the hair at the top of the head with a large clip. Make a part that extends from the outer edge of each eyebrow around the back of the head, and gather the hair above the part in a ponytail at the back of the head. Draw a lock of hair from the ponytail, mist with holding spray, and brush into a flat strip. Wrap the strip around the base of the ponytail to conceal the elastic band.

2. Make a part below the previous part that runs from above the left ear to above the right ear. Brush the hair in this section towards the back of the head and join with the hair in the previous ponytail.

3. Make a ponytail with both groups of hair. Draw a lock of hair from the ponytail, brush into a flat strip, and wrap the strip around the base of the ponytail to conceal the elastic band.

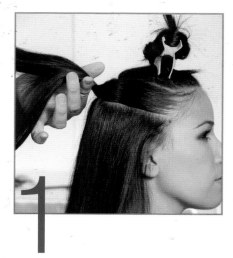

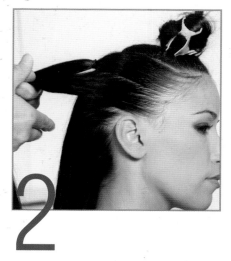

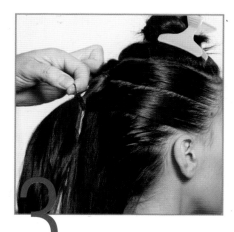

4. Make a part that is 1 inch below the previous part. Gather the hair at the back of the head, join with the previous ponytail, and gather in a third ponytail. Repeat to make a fourth ponytail.

5. Make a fifth and final ponytail at the nape of the neck using the same technique.

6. Release the hair from the clip at the top of the head and backcomb the roots.

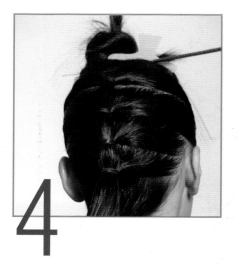

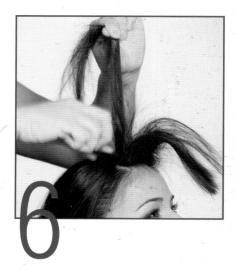

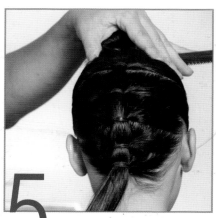

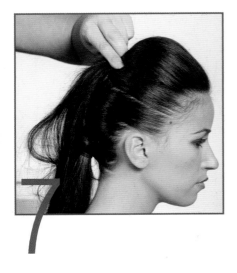

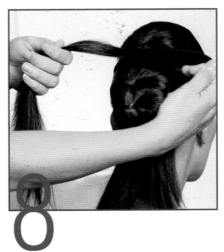

7. Brush the front hair backwards over the backcombed hair and secure with pins just above the top ponytail, leaving the ends loose.

8. Divide the loose ends into two sections.

9. Mist the right section with holding spray and brush into a flat strip. Draw the strip to the right, wrap around a tail comb, then draw towards the left.

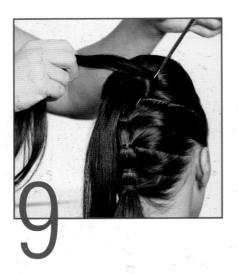

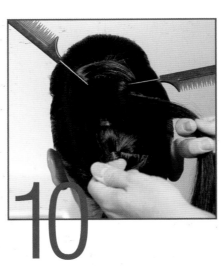

10. Curve the strip in an arc over the top of the ponytail. Support with a tail comb and draw downwards to join this section of hair with the section on the left side. Draw the sections downwards on a diagonal towards the right side of the ponytail.

11. Bring the hair over a tail comb and change directions, drawing the hair downwards and towards the left. Continue in this manner, drawing the hair downwards in a zigzag.

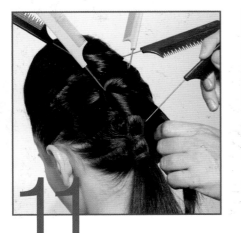

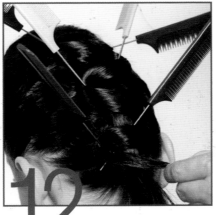

12. Make an effort to conceal the top of each ponytail as you zigzag your way down the back of the head until the nape of the neck.

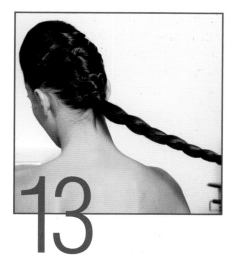

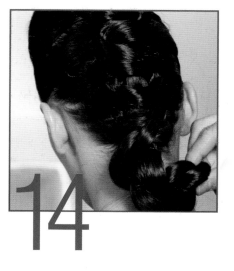

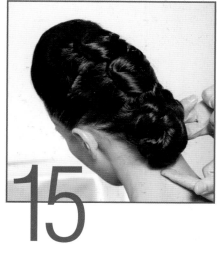

13. Divide the hair in the bottom ponytail into two sections. Twist the sections together to form a rope.

14. Fold the rope in half and roll inwards.

15. Secure with a hairpin at the nape of the neck.

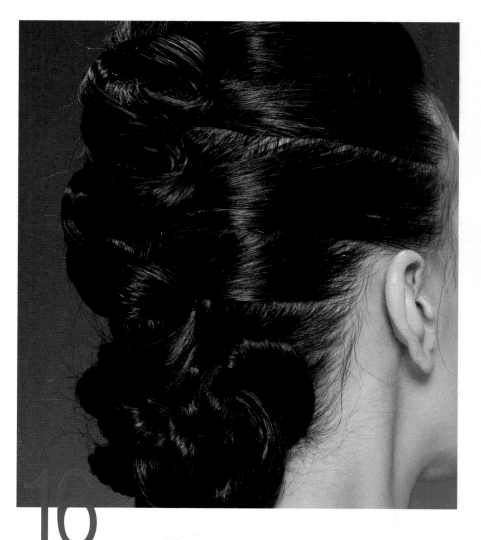

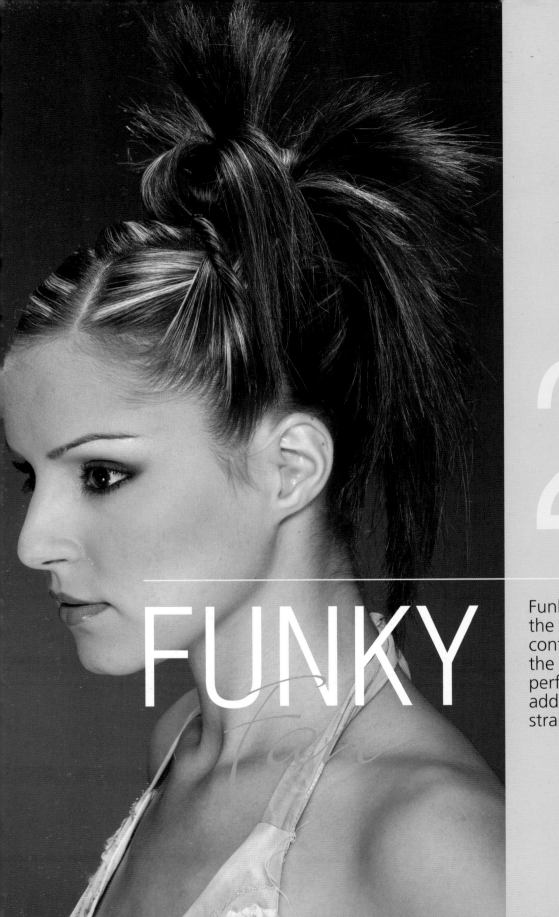

FUNKY

20

Funky and carefree, the loops in this style contrast nicely with the straight ends—a perfect design for adding spunk to straight hair.

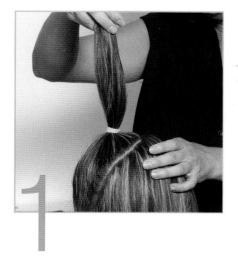

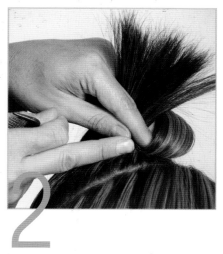

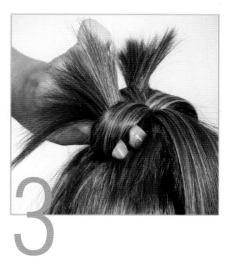

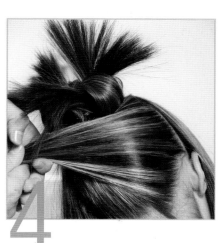

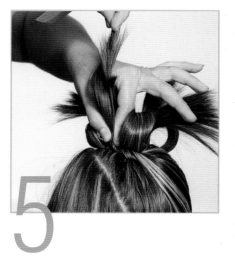

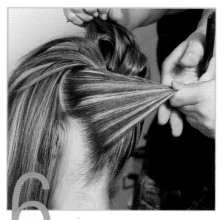

1. Wash and blow dry hair straight. Make a rectangular part at the back of the head that extends from the crown to the nape of the neck. Gather the hair in this section in a high ponytail.

2. Divide the ponytail into four sections. Roll the front section forwards into a loop. Secure the loop near the base of the ponytail, leaving the ends loose.

3. Roll the back section backwards into a loop, and secure near the base of the ponytail, leaving the ends loose. Repeat with the remaining sections of the ponytail, making loops that face the left and right sides.

4. Make a part from the crown to the right ear. Brush the hair behind the part backwards and upwards.

5. Twist the hair upwards and draw it behind the ponytail and to the left side. Secure near the base of the ponytail, leaving the ends loose.

6. Repeat on the other side of the head, making a part from the crown to the left ear, and brushing the hair backwards and upwards.

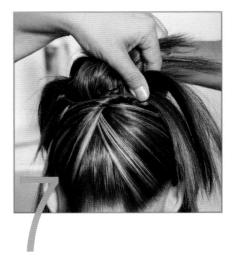

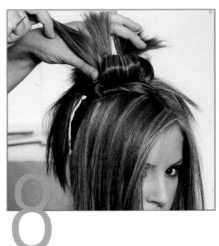

7. Twist the hair upwards and draw it behind the ponytail and to the right side. Secure near the base of the ponytail, leaving the ends loose. Create an envelope of hair with these two sections at the back of the head.

8. Move to the front hair, making a left side part. Gather hair from a 1-inch section on the right side of the part, in front of the ponytail. Twist the hair upwards and backwards. Secure with pins on the right side of the ponytail, leaving the ends loose.

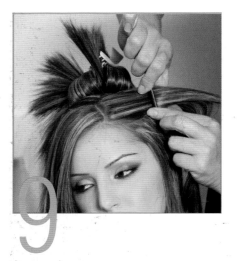

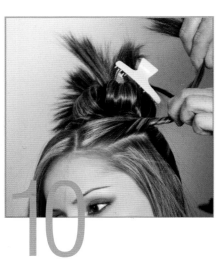

9. Make a diagonal part on the left side of the part.

10. Brush the hair in this section backwards and twist inwards.

11. Secure the hair near the back of the head, to the right of the ponytail, leaving the ends loose.

12. Brush the remaining hair on the front left side and twist upwards. Secure near the front of the ponytail, leaving the ends loose.

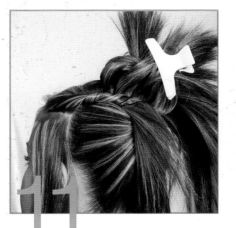

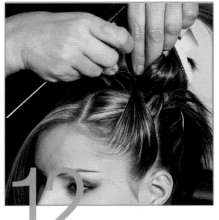

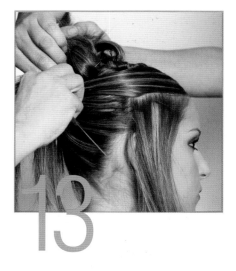

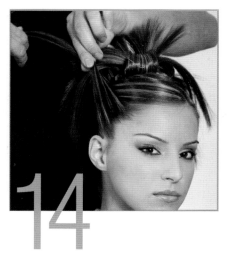

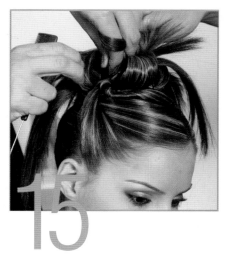

13. Divide the hair on the right side of the part into top and bottom sections. Brush the top section backwards and secure with pins at the back of the head, leaving the ends loose.

14. Brush the remaining section backwards and upwards.

15. Twist the hair forwards and secure with pins between the loops, leaving the ends loose.

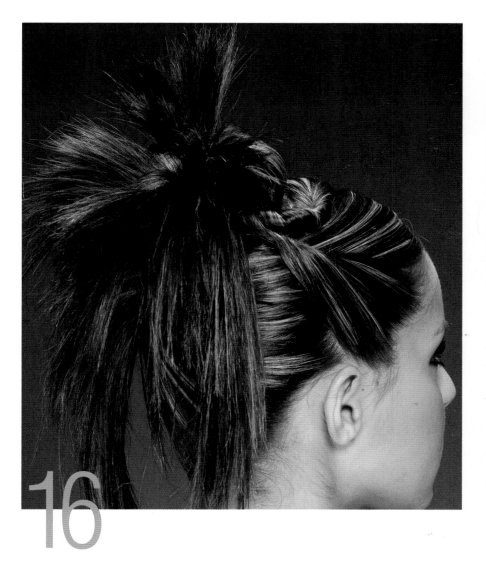

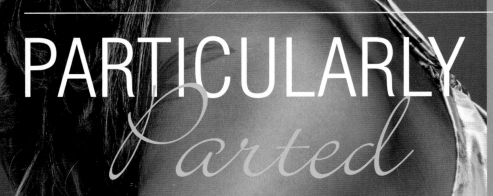

PARTICULARLY
Parted

21

The parts are particularly noticeable in this style, so make sure you use a steady hand and a fine tail comb to make them.

1. Wash and blow dry hair wavy. Make a part from the crown to the right ear. Make another part from the crown to the nape of the neck. Gather the hair between these two parts in a low ponytail behind the right ear.

2. Fold the ponytail upwards and secure with bobby pins, leaving the ends loose.

3. Make a diagonal part on the left side of the head and twist the hair backwards. Secure with pins above the ponytail.

4. Make a part on the left side of the crown and mist with holding spray.

5. Twist the hair upwards and towards the ponytail. Secure with an X of bobby pins, leaving the ends loose.

6. Make a horizontal part about 2 inches below this part and brush the hair towards the right side. Twist the hair upwards and secure with a bobby pin, leaving the ends loose.

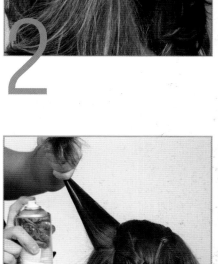

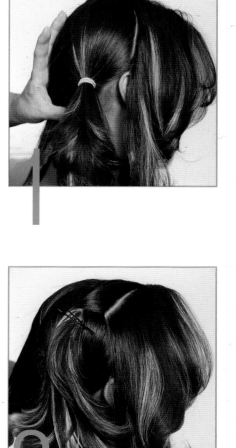

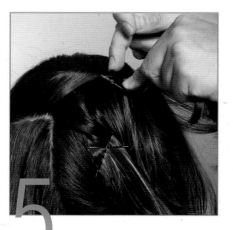

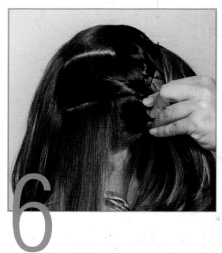

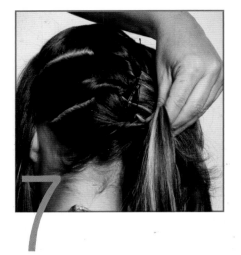

7

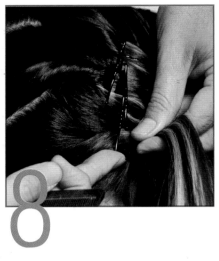

8

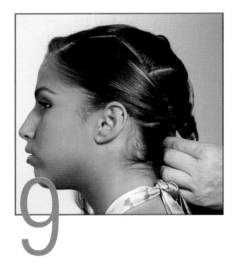

9

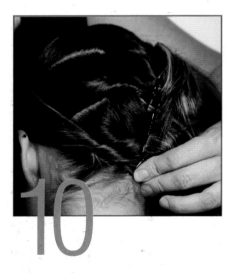

10

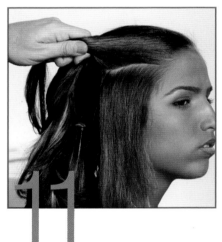

11

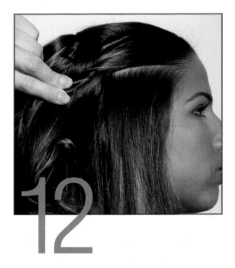

12

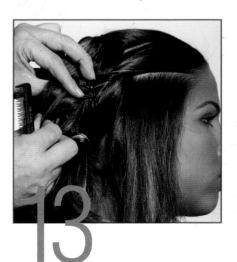

13

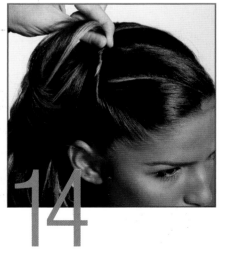

14

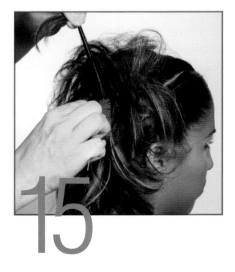

15

7. Repeat with the bottom section of hair, brushing it towards the right and twisting it upwards.

8. Secure the hair with pins, leaving the ends loose.

9. Brush the remaining section of hair on the left side of the head downwards and backwards.

10. Twist the hair upwards and draw it towards the left side of the head. Secure with pins under the pins on the right side of the head, leaving the ends loose.

11. Divide the hair on the front right side into top and bottom sections.

12. Twist the top section upwards and draw towards the back of the head.

13. Secure with an X of bobby pins, leaving the ends loose.

14. Brush the remaining hair and twist inwards and upwards to cover the pins. Secure with a bobby pin, leaving the ends loose.

15. Backcomb the loose ends at the back of the head to the roots to add volume.

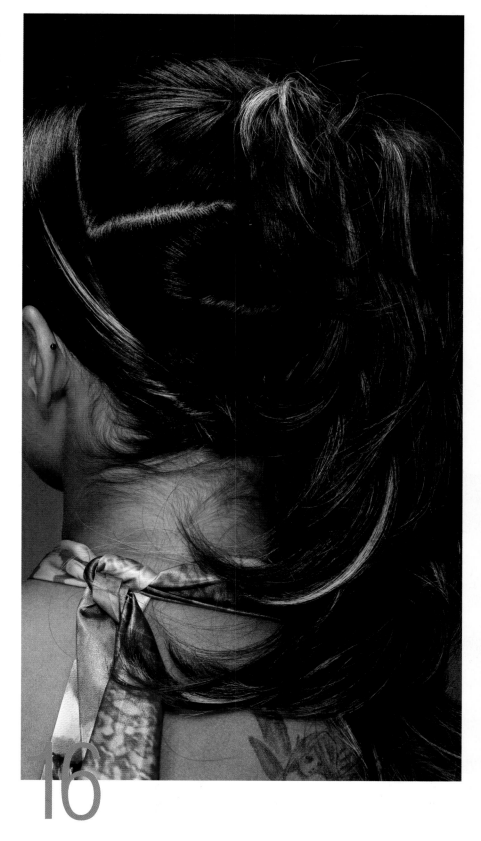

16

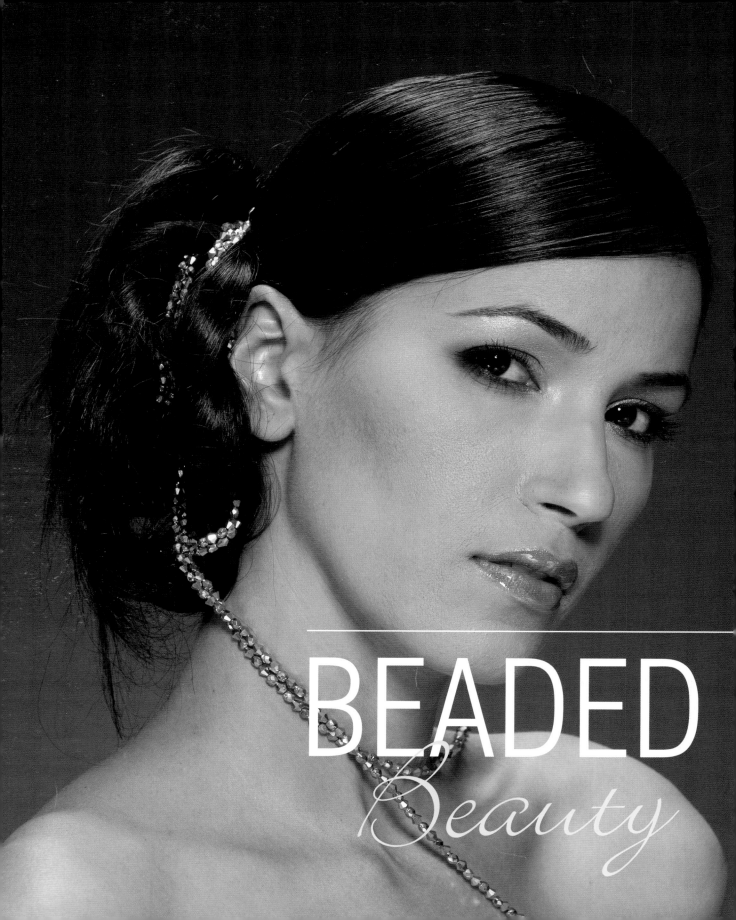

BEADED *Beauty*

22

Show off a favorite beaded necklace with this hairstyle. Wrap any excess necklace around the shoulders and neck to finish the look.

1. Wash and blow dry hair straight. Divide the hair into front and back sections with a part that extends from ear to ear over the crown. Gather the front section in a clip. Gather the back section in a low ponytail on the right side. Draw a lock of hair from the ponytail, mist with holding spray, and brush into a flat strip. Wrap around the base of the ponytail to conceal the elastic band. Select a long beaded necklace.

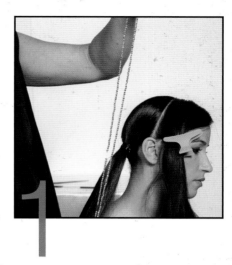

2. Attach the necklace at the base of the ponytail with a hairpin. Divide the ponytail into two sections.

3. Plait a braid using the two sections of the ponytail and the necklace.

4. Secure the braid with an elastic band. Fold the braid in half, drawing the end up behind the right ear.

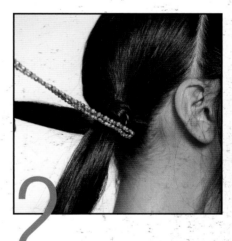

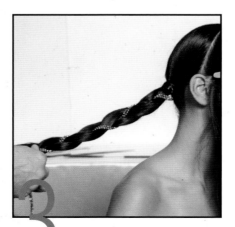

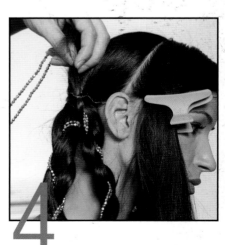

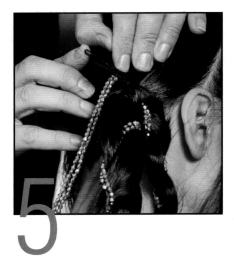

5

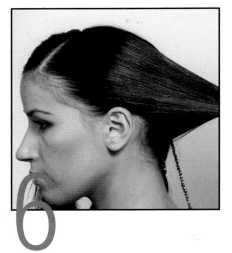

6

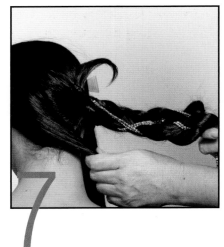

7

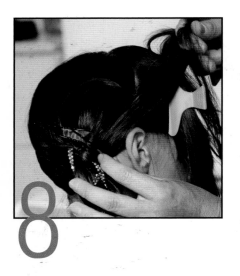

8

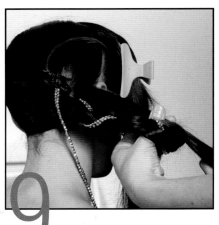

9

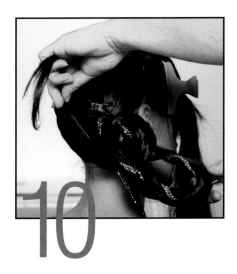

10

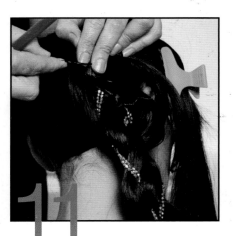

11

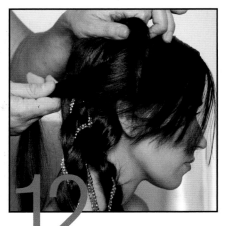

12

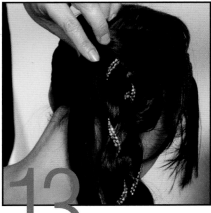

13

5. Secure the braid with a hairpin, leaving the ends loose.

6. Make a left side part in the front hair and brush the hair to the left of the part downwards and backwards.

7. Draw the hair under the braid.

8. Now draw the hair upwards over the right ear. Secure the hair close to the base of the braid, leaving the ends loose.

9. Draw the ends of the hair downwards, over the bottom of the braid, and through the loop of the braid.

10. Draw the hair under the top of the braid, and upwards towards the back of the head.

11. Secure the hair just above the top of the braid, leaving the ends loose.

12. Brush the hair to the right of the part backwards and down-wards, drawing it over the end of the braid to conceal it.

13. Secure with hairpins at the back of the head, leaving the ends loose.

14. Brush the remaining hair at the front of the head backwards. Tuck the hair using a tail comb and mist with holding spray.

15. Elegantly wrap any excess necklace around the neck and shoulders.

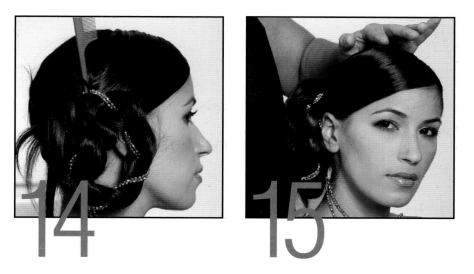

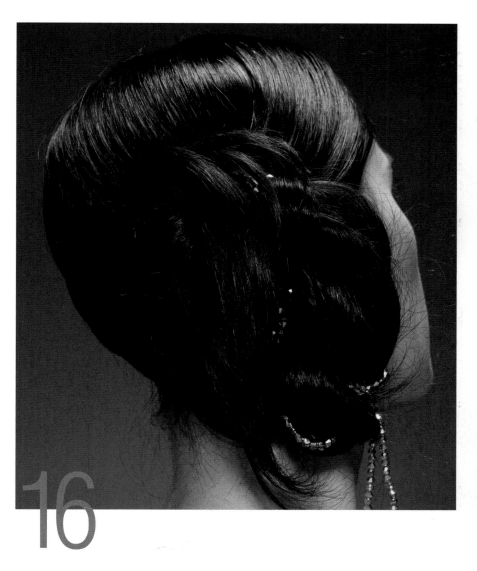

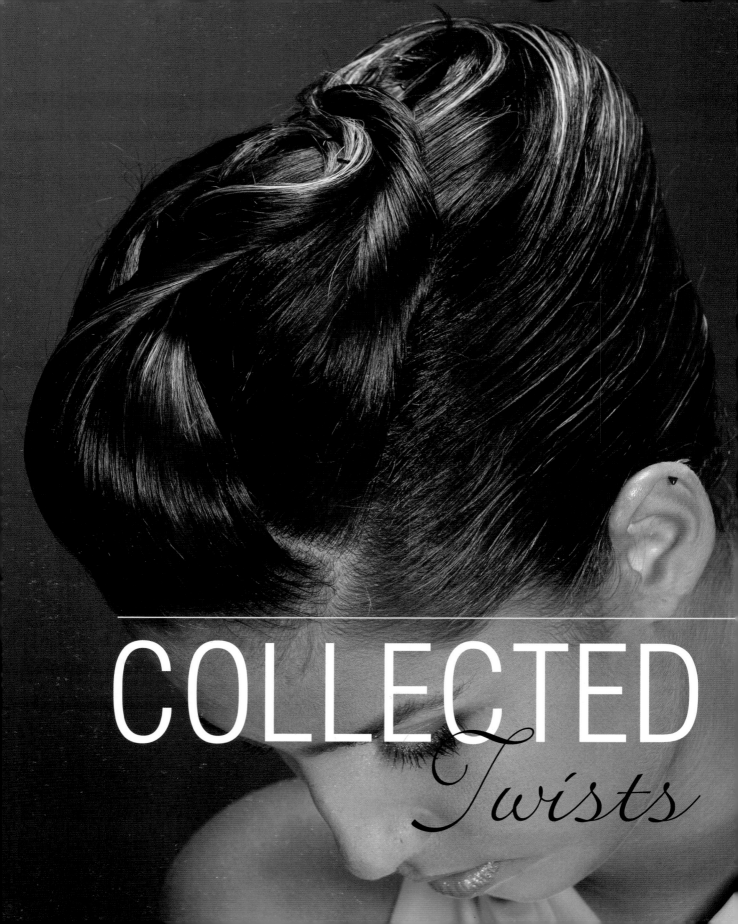

COLLECTED
Twists

23

This elegant assortment of twists includes a large twist at the back of the head, two coils at the top, and a half-twist at the front.

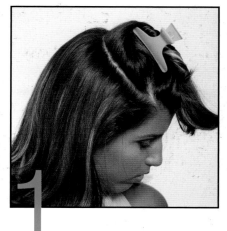

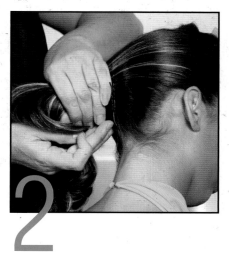

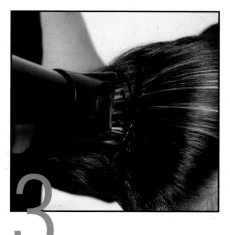

1. Wash and blow dry hair wavy. Gather the hair at the top of the head in a clip.

2. Brush the hair on the right side of the head backwards. Secure with a vertical seam of pins at the back of the head.

3. Mist with holding spray and blow dry on medium heat.

4. Brush the hair on the left side of the head backwards and upwards.

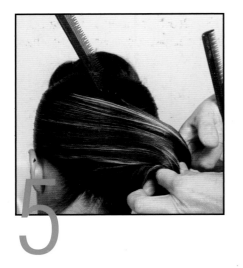

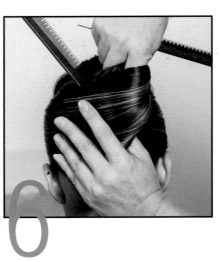

5. Make a large twist by rolling the hair inwards over two fingers.

6. Draw the twisted hair upwards.

7. Secure the twist with bobby pins.

8. Insert hairpins along the length of the twist to secure.

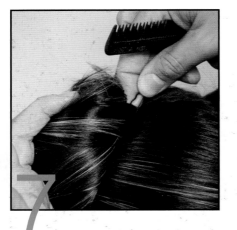

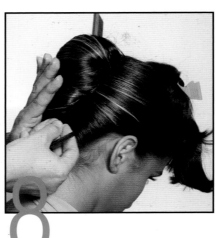

9. Take a section of hair from the top of the head, to the right of the crown. Brush the hair backwards and towards the left side of the head. Mist with holding spray.

10. Coil the hair to make a flat Figure 6 and secure with hairpins at the top of the large twist.

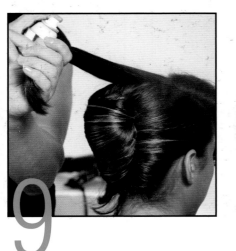

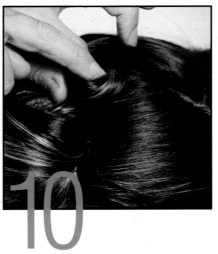

11. Take a section of hair from the left side of the crown. Brush it backwards and towards the right side of the head. Mist with holding spray.

12. Coil the hair tightly to make a flat Figure 6. Tuck into the middle of the previous Figure 6, and secure with hairpins.

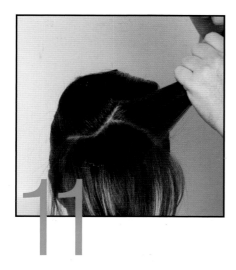

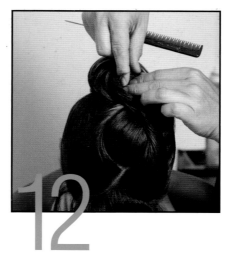

13. Brush the bangs upwards and backwards, twisting the hair gently.

14. Coil the end of the bangs and secure with hairpins on the top of the head.

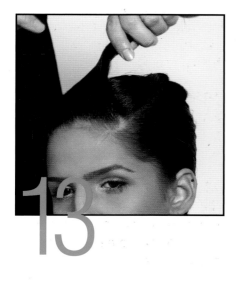

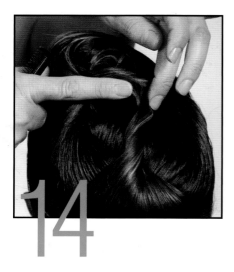

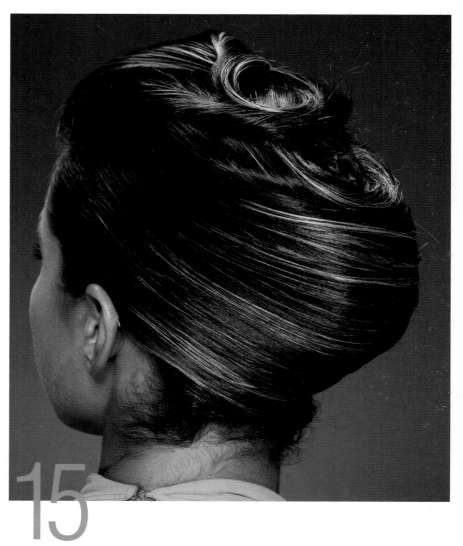

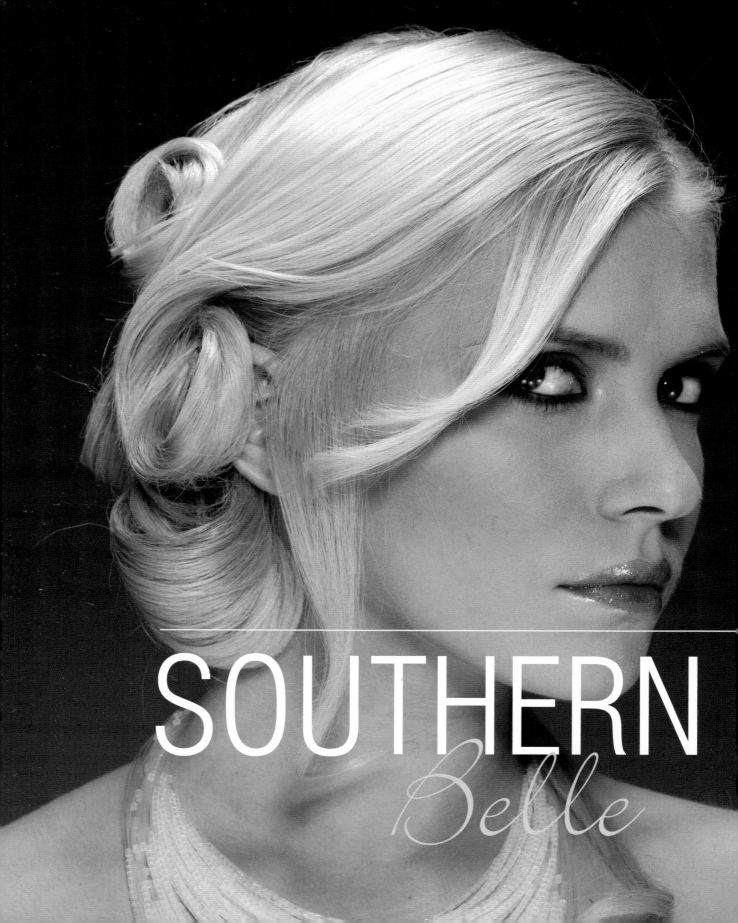

SOUTHERN *Belle*

1. Wash and blow dry hair wavy, using a round brush to add volume.

2. Make a part from the crown to the top of the right ear. Gather the hair in this section in a large clip.

3. Make another part that extends from the crown to the nape of the neck, marking off a triangular section that is about 2 inches wide at its base. Gather the hair in a low ponytail at the nape of the neck.

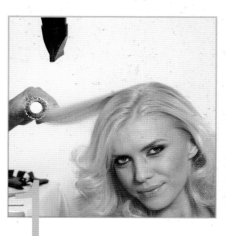

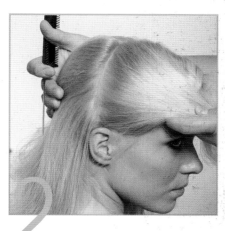

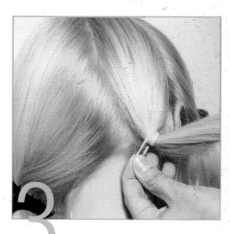

24

This flowing design features six large, graceful curls that are pinned to the right side of the head. Leaving a few wisps at the front increases the romance.

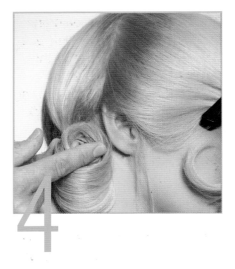

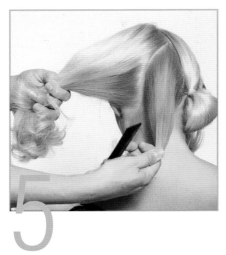

4. Coil the hair forwards and upwards into a flat Figure 6. Secure with a hairpin under the base of the ponytail.

5. Make a part at the back of the head to mark off a triangular section of hair that is 1 1/2 inches wide at its base.

6. Brush the hair in this section towards the ponytail at the right.

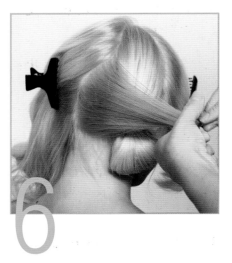

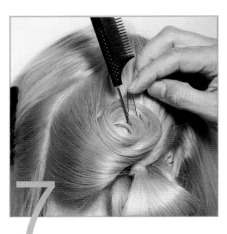

7. Coil the hair upwards into a flat Figure 6 and secure with hairpins.

8. Move leftwards at the back of the head and make another part to mark off another section of hair, this one a little larger than the previous section.

9. Brush the hair into a flat strip. Coil inwards and upwards into a flat Figure 6. Secure the hair above the previous flat Figure 6 with hairpins.

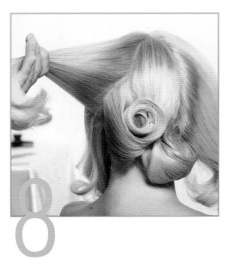

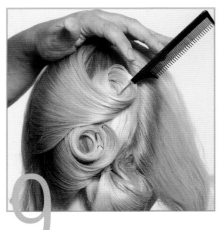

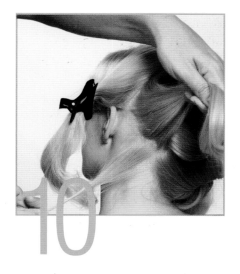

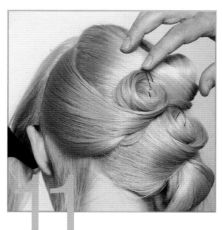

10. Move leftwards again and make a part behind the left ear. Gather the hair in front of the part in a clip. Brush the hair behind the part upwards, leaving a lock of hair loose at the neck.

11. Coil this section upwards into a flat Figure 6 and secure with a hairpin at the back of the head.

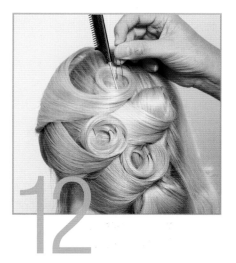

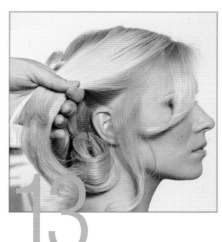

12. Brush the front hair on the left side of the head backwards. Coil into a flat Figure 6 and secure with hairpins at the back of the head.

13. Brush the front hair on the right side backwards. Leave a few locks of hair loose at the face, and brush the rest backwards and downwards.

14. Coil the hair into a flat Figure 6 and secure with hairpins.

15. Mist with finishing spray.

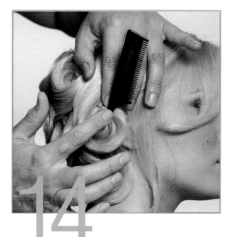

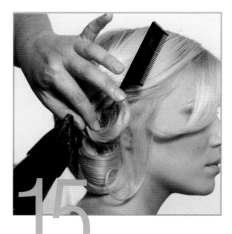

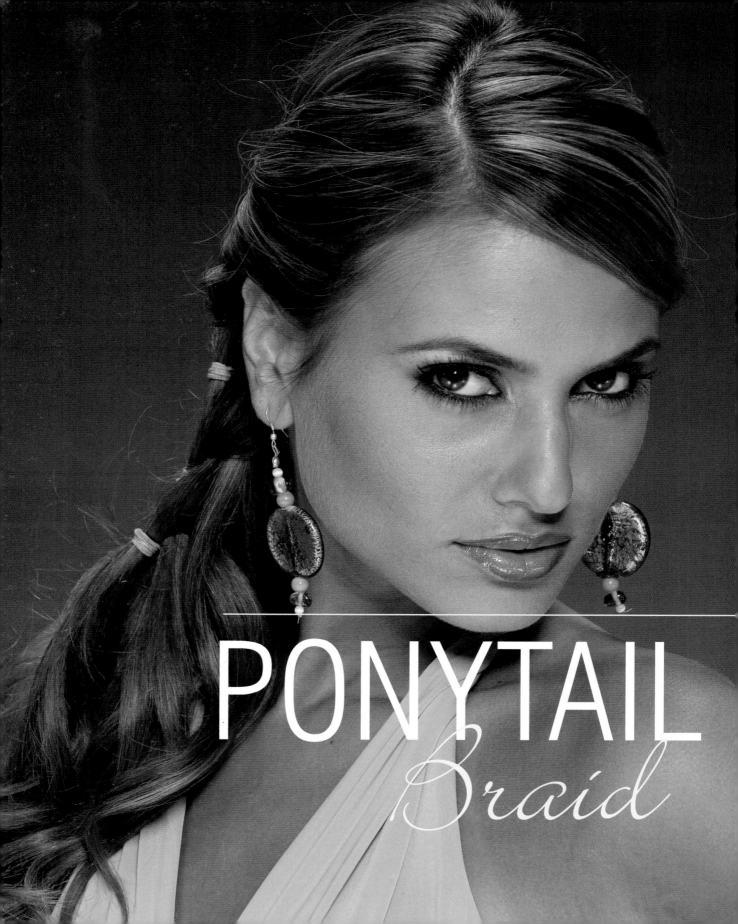

PONYTAIL
Braid

1. Wash and blow dry hair. Curl the ends into ringlets with a curling iron, then brush out with a round brush. Make a right side part.

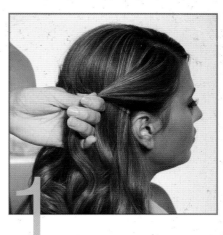

2. Gather a section of hair that extends from the part to the right ear. Gather a similar section of hair from the part to the left ear. Gather the two sections together at the back of the head, behind the right ear.

3. Join the two sections in a ponytail that is just above the right ear.

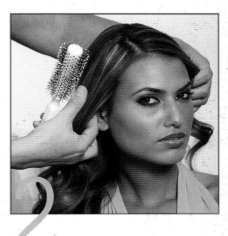

25

Simply select elastic bands that complement your outfit to add a splash of color to your hair.

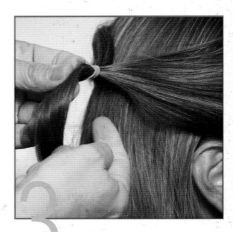

4. Gather hair from a section of hair behind the right ear.

5. Gather a similar section of hair from behind the left ear and draw the two sections of hair together at the back of the head, over the hair extending from the previous ponytail, and about 2 inches below it. Join in a second ponytail.

6. Gather sections of hair from the right and left sides of the head.

7. Join the sections in a ponytail over the hair in the previous ponytail, and about 2 inches below it. Draw this ponytail a little bit towards the right.

8. Repeat again, gathering sections of hair from both sides of the head, and joining them in a ponytail that is 2 inches below the previous ponytail, and slightly towards the right. Mist with holding spray as necessary.

9. Repeat to make a fourth ponytail.

10. Continue in this manner, making a braid of ponytails, until you reach the neck.

11. In this manner, make an exterior braid of ponytails.

12. Mist with finishing spray.

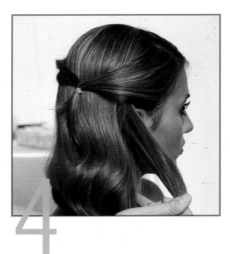
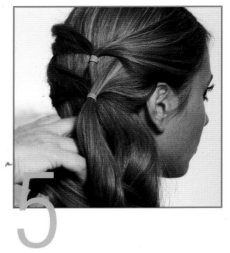
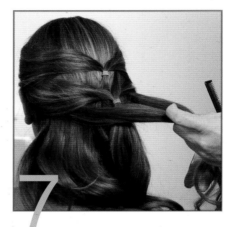
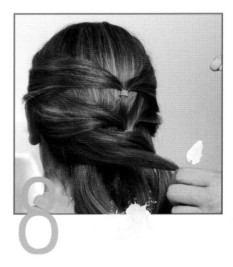
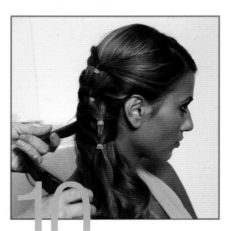
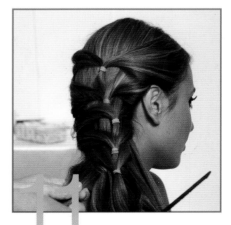

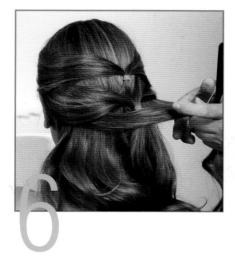

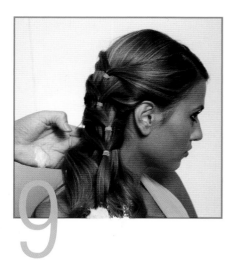

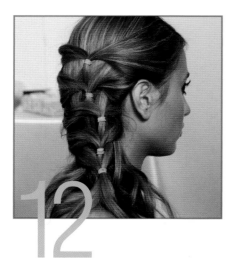

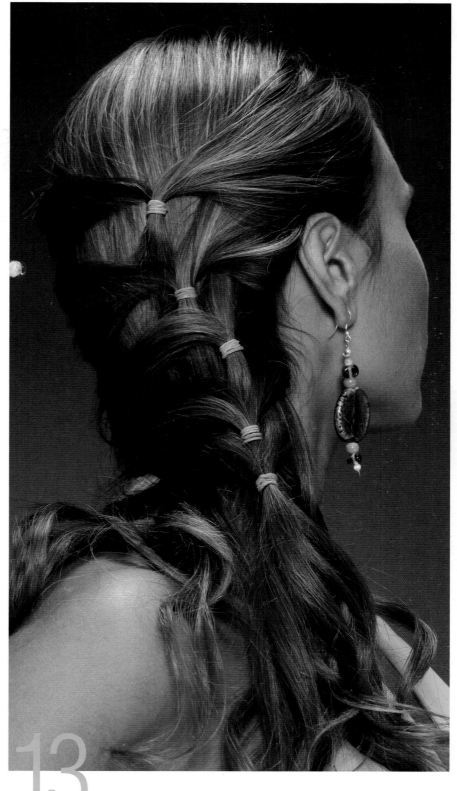

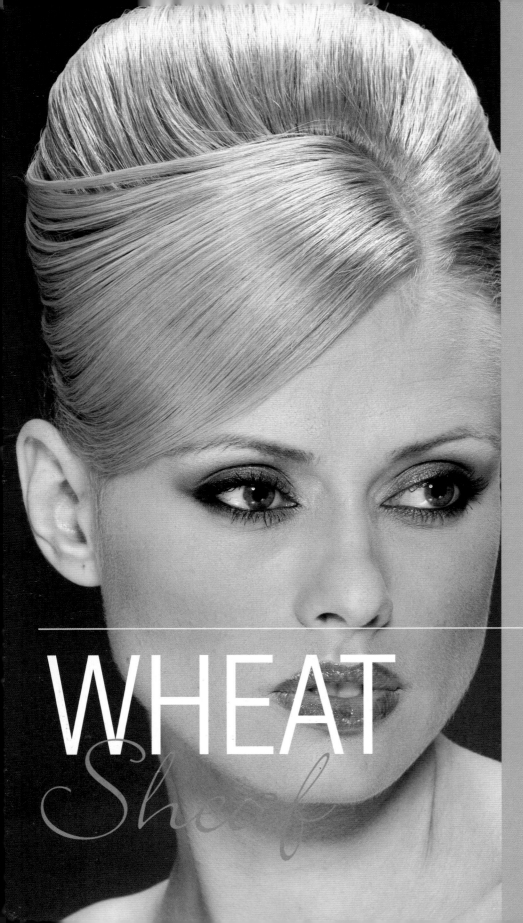

WHEAT
Sheaf

26

Weaving the hair carefully with a tail comb creates a pattern that resembles a wheat sheaf just before harvesting.

1. Wash and blow dry hair straight. Make a left side part to the crown. Make a part from the crown to the top of the right ear and gather the hair in this section in a large clip. Backcomb a triangular section of hair behind the part to make a spongy base.

2. Brush the backcombed hair forwards and secure with a seam of pins.

3. Make a diagonal part to the right of the spongy base. Brush the hair into a flat strip and mist with holding spray. Draw upwards and over to the left side of the spongy base.

4. Secure the hair with bobby pins at the left side of the spongy base. Insert the pins so that they are in line with the previous pins. Make a diagonal part on the left side of the spongy base. Brush the hair into a flat strip, mist with holding spray, and draw to the right of the spongy base.

5. Brush the remaining hair on the right side of the spongy base backwards and upwards.

6. Draw this hair over the hair that was drawn from the left side, and secure with pins on the left side of the spongy base, making an X of hair at the back of the head. Repeat with the remaining hair on the left side of the spongy base.

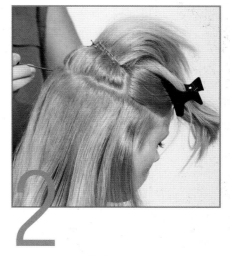

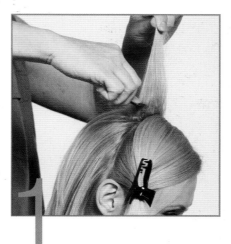

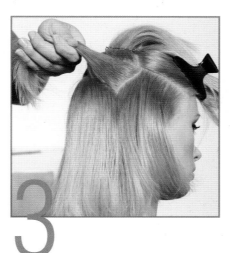

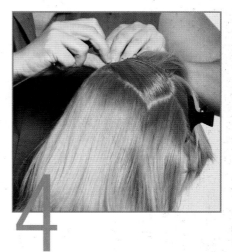

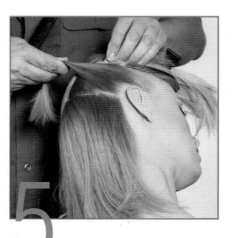

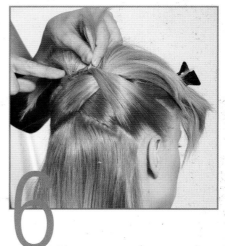

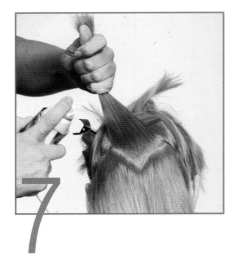

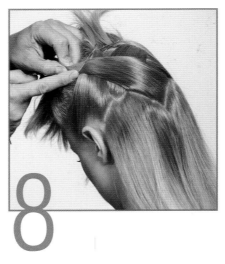

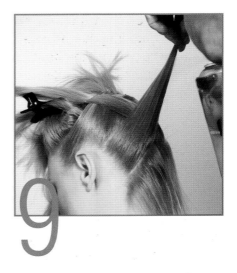

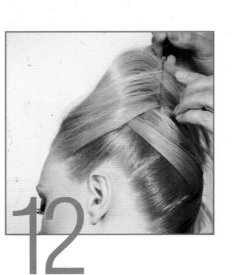

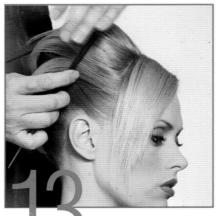

7. Make a triangular part at the back of the head, below the X of hair. Mist with holding spray and brush the hair upwards and to the left.

8. Secure this hair with a bobby pin over the section of hair that was drawn to the right, to make another X of hair at the back of the head.

9. Gather a 1-inch section of hair below the left ear. Brush the hair into a flat strip, mist with holding spray, and draw upwards towards the right side of the head. Secure with bobby pins.

10. Repeat on the other side of the head, gathering hair from a similar section below the right ear. Brush the hair into a flat strip, mist with holding spray, and draw upwards and towards the left side of the head. Secure with bobby pins.

11. Brush the last section of hair upwards from the nape of the neck and draw over to the right side of the head, creating a sheaf-like pattern at the back of the head.

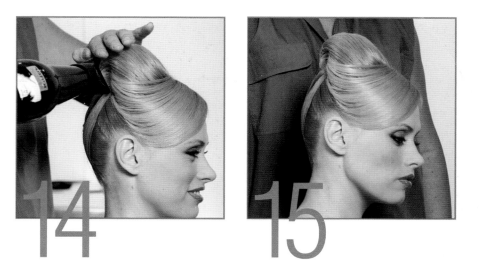

12. Brush the hair at the front left side of the head backwards and over the seam of pins at the top of the sheaf pattern, to conceal it.

13. Divide the hair on the front right side into front and back sections. Brush the hair in the back section backwards and over the seam of pins, adding height to the top of the hair-style. Secure in place with hairpins.

14. Brush the front section of hair so that it sweeps over the brow and flows upwards towards the back of the head. Mist with holding spray, secure with hairpins, and blow dry on medium heat.

15. Tuck any stray hairs into place and mist with finishing spray.

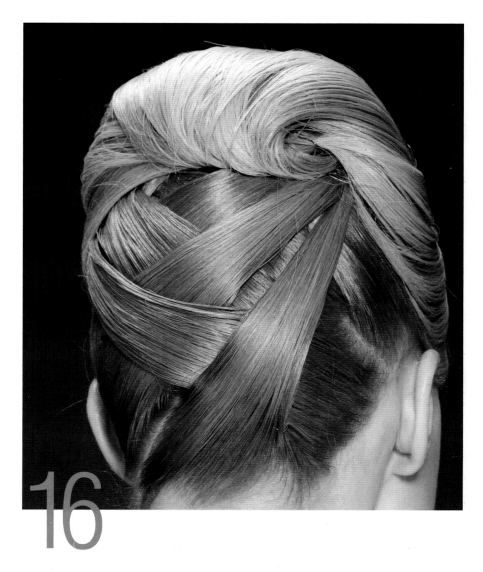

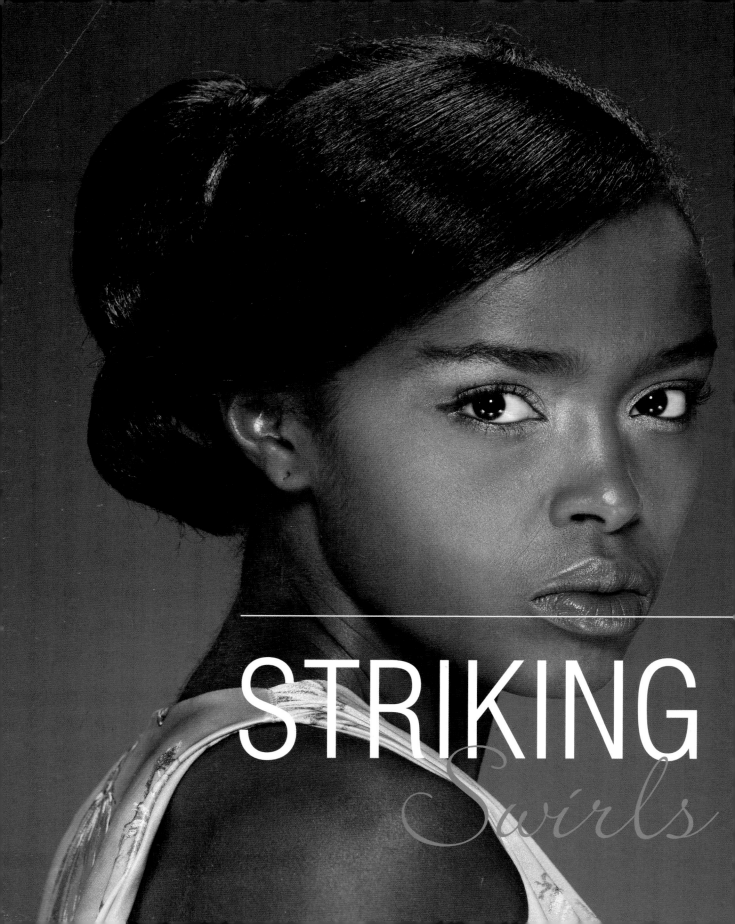

STRIKING *Swirls*

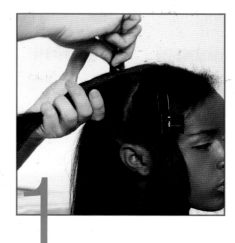

1. Wash and blow dry hair straight. Divide the hair into front and back sections with a part that extends from ear to ear over the crown. Make a left side part in the front hair and gather the hair on either side of the part in clips.

2. Make a triangular part from the crown to the right ear. Gather the hair in this section in a ponytail.

3. Gather the remaining hair in a low ponytail on the right side of the head.

4. Brush the bottom ponytail into a flat strip. Mist with holding spray and blow dry. Roll the hair downwards over two fingers to form a large loop. Tuck the ends of the hair into the loop as you roll it.

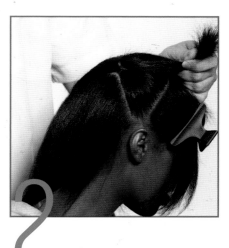

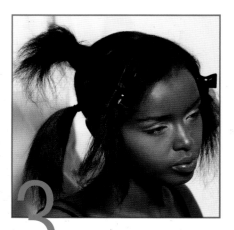

27

This hairstyle features a striking combination. The front is smooth and sleek; the back features gentle rolls and curls.

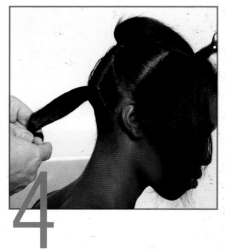

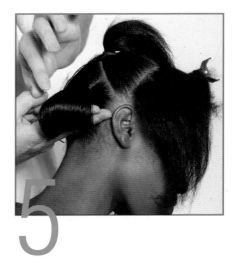

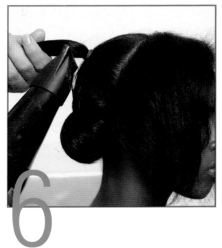

5. Secure the loop to the head with hairpins at either side.

6. Brush the top ponytail into a flat strip. Mist with holding spray and blow dry.

7. Draw the ponytail downwards and insert the ends into the loop. Secure with pins.

8. Release the front hair from the clips. Brush the hair on the right side downwards and towards the right ear.

9. Twist the hair upwards after it passes the ear, using a tail comb for support.

10. Wrap the ends of the hair around the top ponytail and secure with bobby pins. Mist with holding spray, and remove the tail comb.

11. Brush the hair on the front left side of the head upwards and backwards.

12. Draw the hair towards the top ponytail.

13. Tuck the ends of the hair into the ponytail, using a tail comb for support. Secure with a hairpin, mist with holding spray, and remove the tail comb.

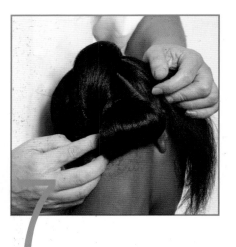

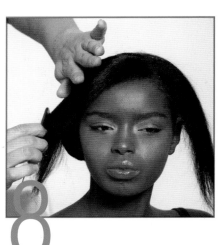

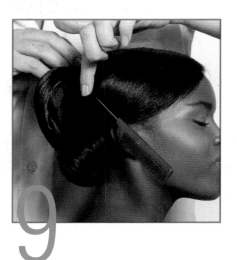

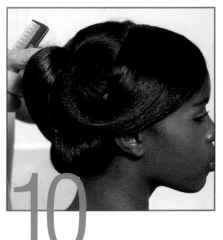

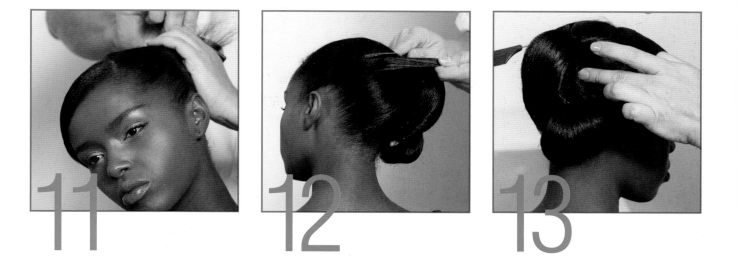

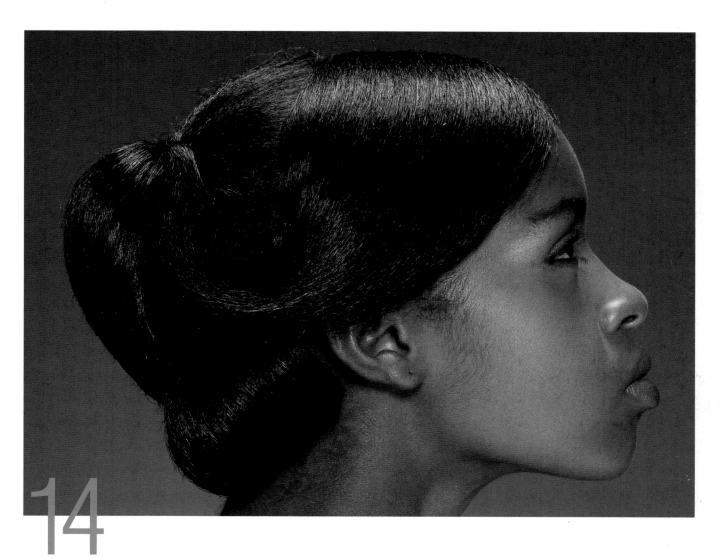

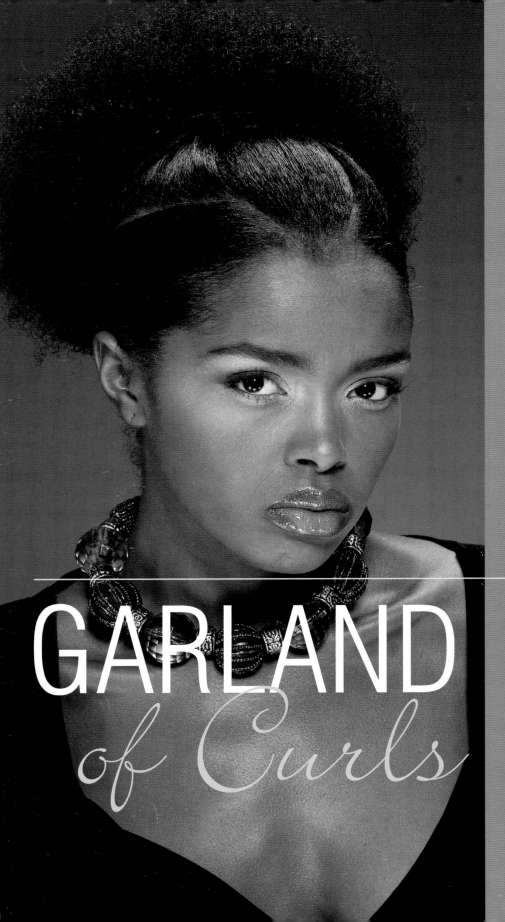

28

GARLAND
of Curls

Makes the most out of a curly mane of hair by setting off curls at the back with a tightly combed front.

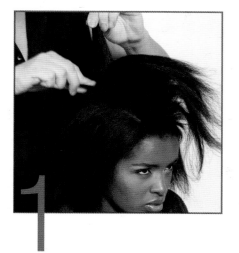

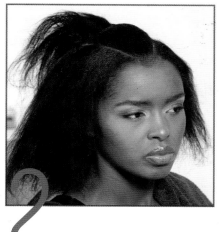

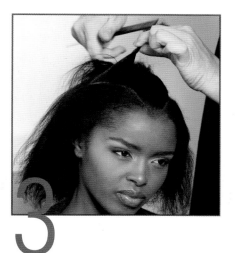

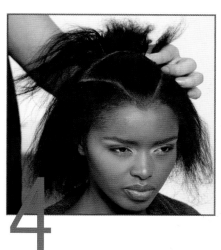

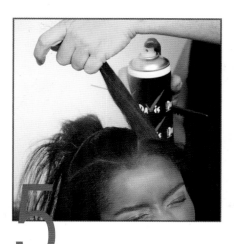

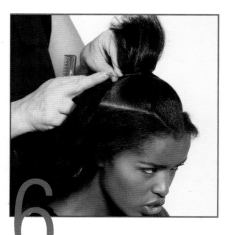

1. Wash and blow dry hair straight. Make a triangular part from the brow to the crown that peaks at the brow. Backcomb the hair in the triangle.

2. Brush the top of the back-combed hair backwards and secure with a seam of pins at the base of the triangle to make a spongy triangular base.

3. Take a section of hair along the right of the triangle. Mist with holding spray and twist upwards.

4. Draw the hair backwards to the opposite side of the triangle and secure near the seam of pins.

5. Take a section of hair along the left side of the triangle. Mist with holding spray, twist it upwards, and draw it backwards to the opposite side of the triangle.

6. Secure near the seam of pins.

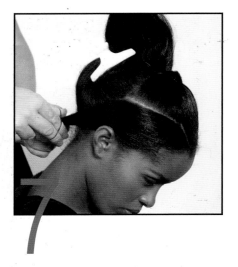

7

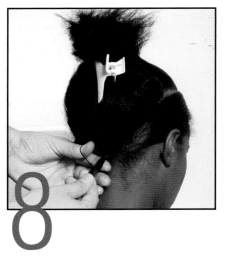

8

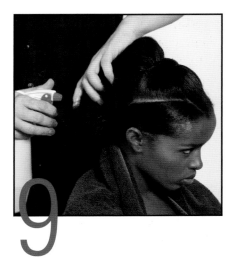

9

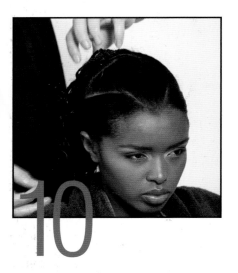

10

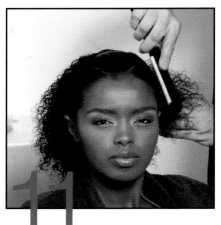

11

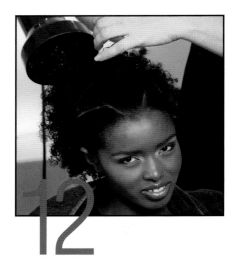

12

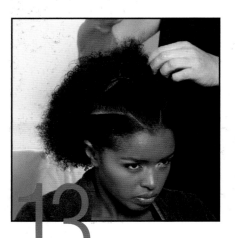

13

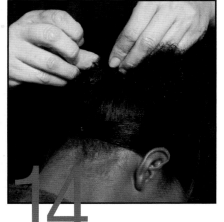

14

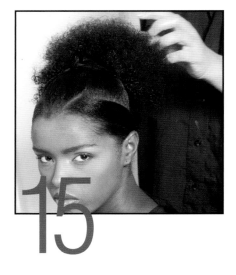

15

7. Gather the hair in the middle and back of the head with a clip. Mist holding spray on the hair at the sides. Draw firmly downwards and towards the back of the head.

8. Gather the hair from both sides at the back in a low ponytail.

9. Release the hair from the clip and mist with water until very wet.

10. Massage styling gel into the wet hair.

11. Carefully comb the wet hair, taking care not to disturb the hair that has been smoothed backwards.

12. Blow dry the wet hair evenly with a diffuser to bring out the natural curl.

13. Comb with a wide tooth comb to loosen the curls.

14. Brush the hair at the nape of the neck upwards and secure with bobby pins.

15. The final effect should be a round bouquet of curls at the back of the head.

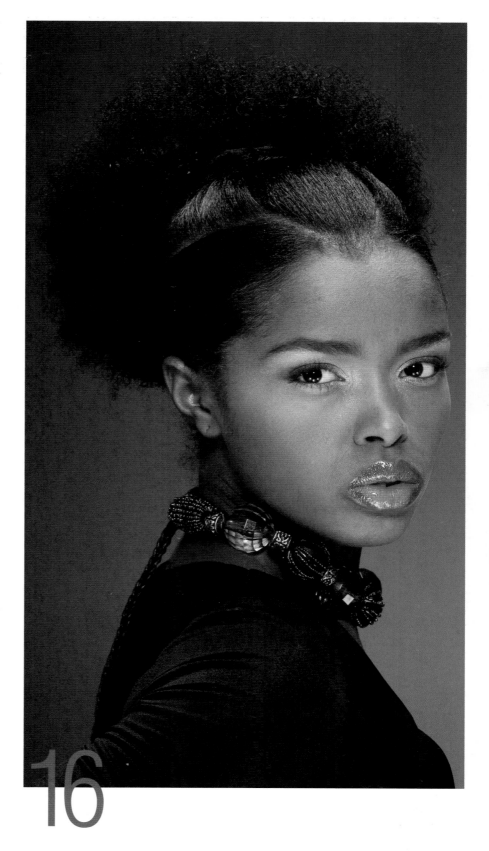

16

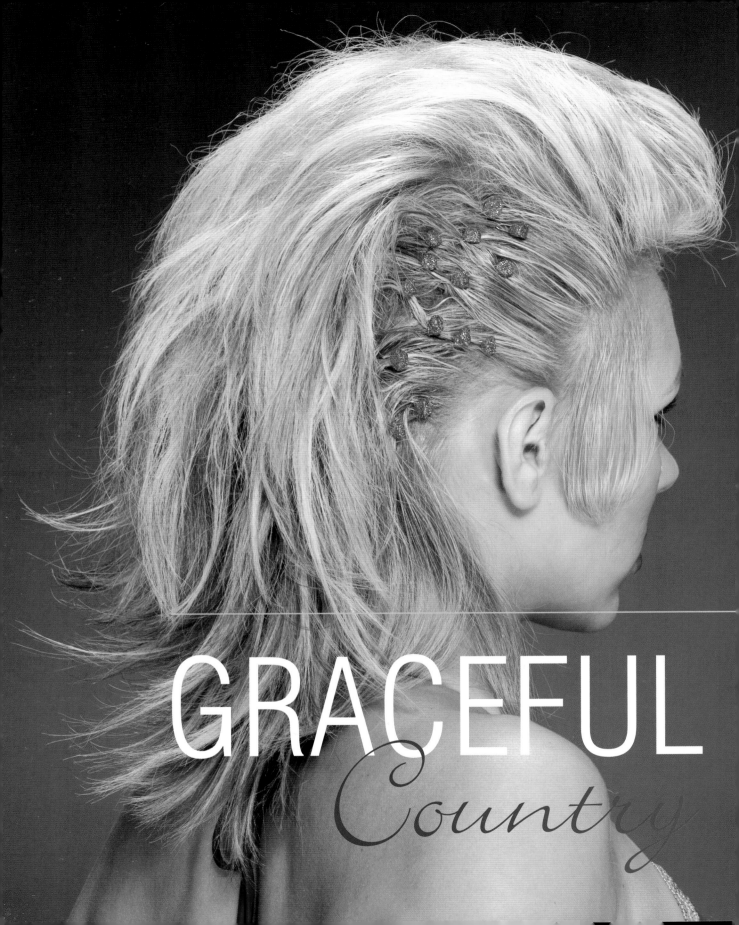

GRACEFUL

Country

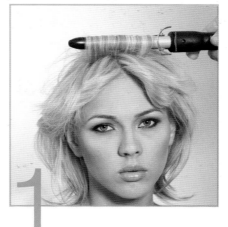

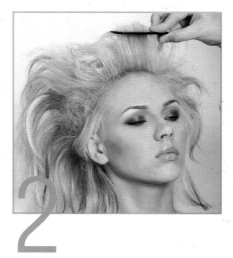

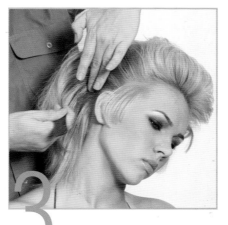

29

This hairstyle won't go unnoticed. Use bold hair accessories for maximum pizzazz.

1. Wash and blow dry hair straight. Curl the hair at the top of the head with a curling iron.

2. Backcomb all of the hair. Brush the hair at the brow upwards.

3. Brush the hair at the sides upwards, drawing out the locks just above the ears.

4. Mist holding spray on the hair at the sides. Start at the top of the hair and move towards the roots, spraying generously and in a straight line.

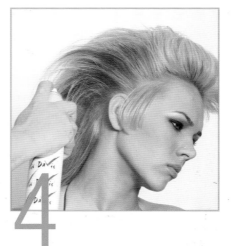

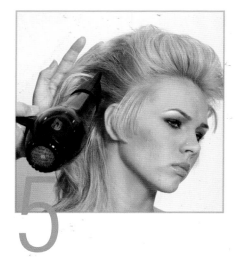

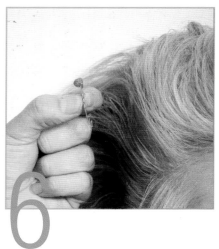

5. Blow dry hair on medium heat until it is completely dry. Take particular care to dry thoroughly at the roots.

6. Select decorative hairpins.

7. Secure the hairpins along the side of the hair to support the hold.

8. Work your way from the front of the head to the back, placing hairpins on both sides of the head.

9. Brush down the locks of hair on either side of the face.

10. Comb out the hair at the back with a wide tooth comb.

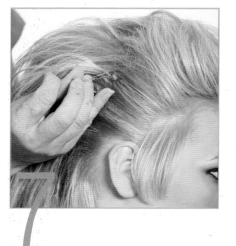

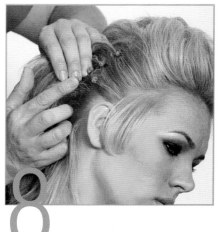

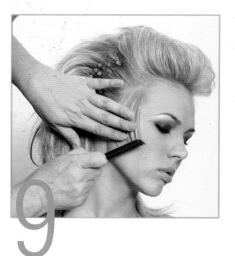

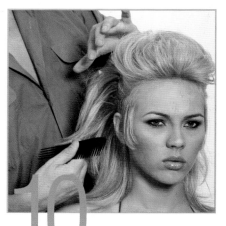

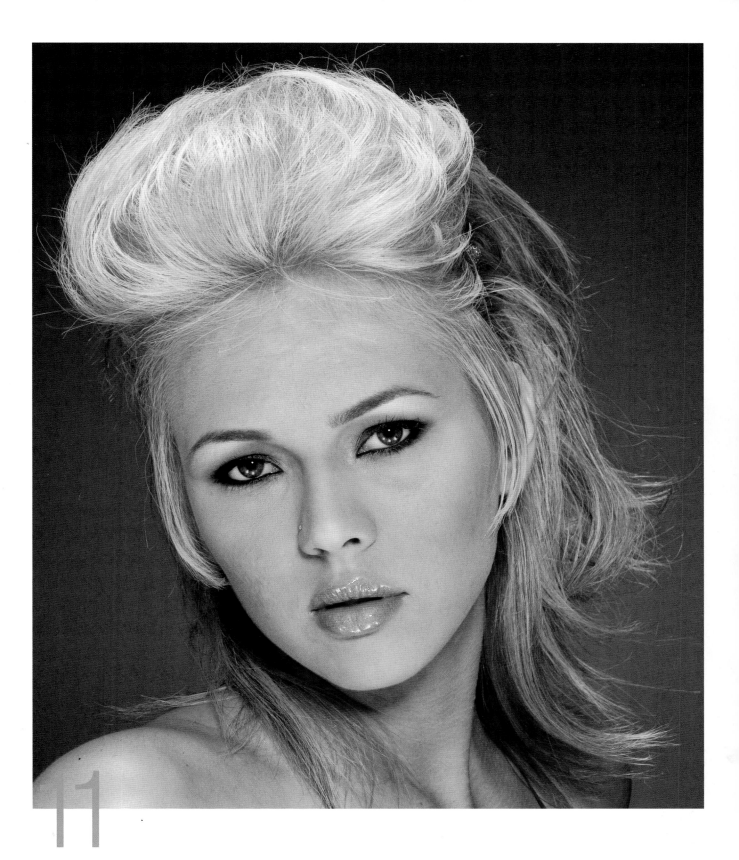

11

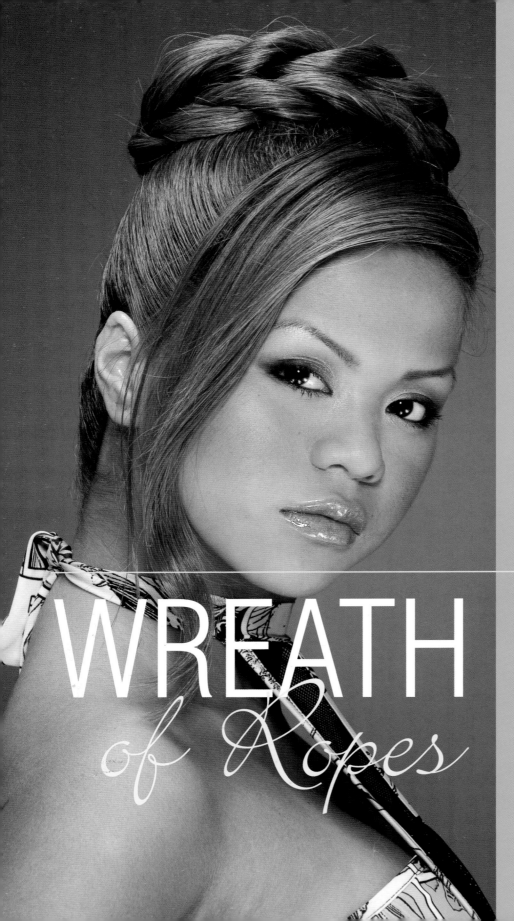

30

WREATH
of Ropes

Look like a modern princess with this wreath of twisted hair. Use a long hair extension to make ropes that are especially thick.

1. Wash hair and blow dry straight. Hold the bangs with a clip. Make a part in the shape of an upside-down V at the back of the head and gather the top hair in a high ponytail.

2. Select a straight hair extension and divide into three sections, so that the middle section is wider than the side sections.

3. Place the extension under the ponytail. Wrap the side sections in an X over the top of the ponytail.

4. Secure the extension to the head with bobby pins.

5. Draw the natural ponytail forwards and divide the main part of the extension into two halves. Divide the right half into two sections. Twist the sections together to form a rope. Repeat with the left half of the extension.

6. Twist the left rope over the front of the ponytail and towards the right.

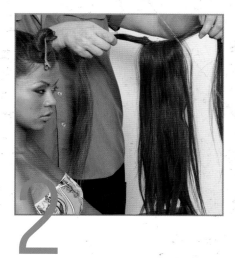

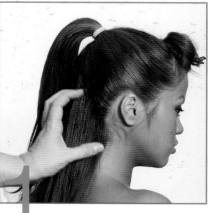

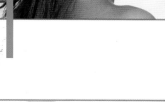

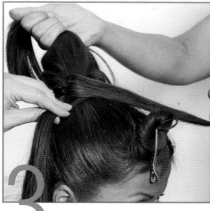

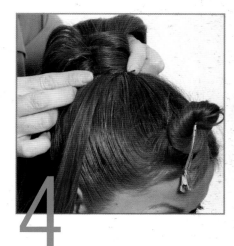

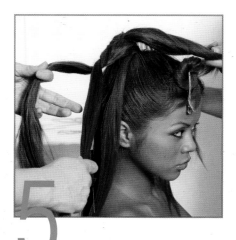

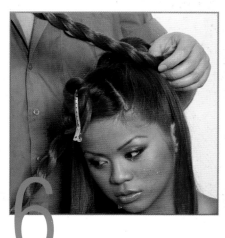

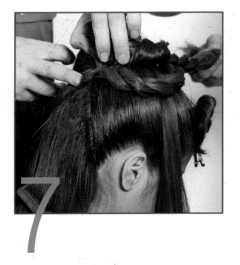

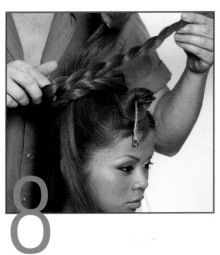

7. Wrap the rope around the back of the ponytail and secure with pins at the top of the V-shaped part.

8. Twist the right rope over the front of the head and towards the left side. Lay this rope on top of the previous rope, and secure with pins at the back of the head, under the ponytail.

9. Brush the natural ponytail into a flat strip and coil inside the wreath of ropes. Use tail combs to secure the coil.

10. Brush the hair below the V-shaped part upwards.

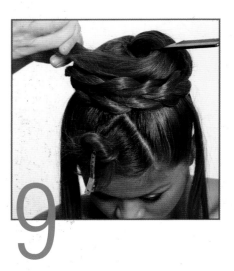

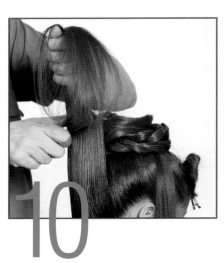

11. Coil the hair into a flat Figure 6 and secure with pins in the middle of the coil.

12. Grasp the loose sections of the extension on either side of the head and twist outwards.

13. Cross the sections at the back of the head in an X under the wreath.

14. Tuck the ends around the wreath and secure with hairpins. Release the bangs and brush to the right.

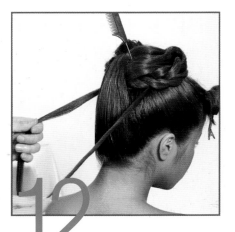

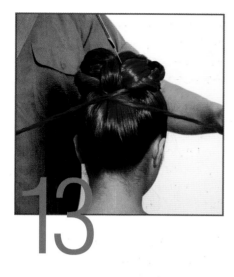

13

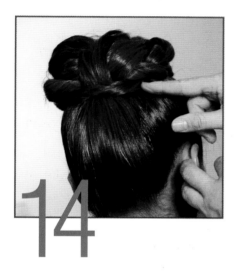

14

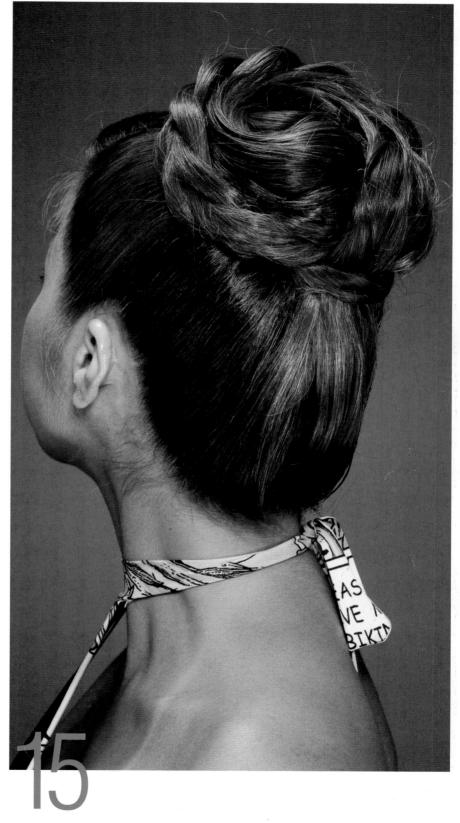

15

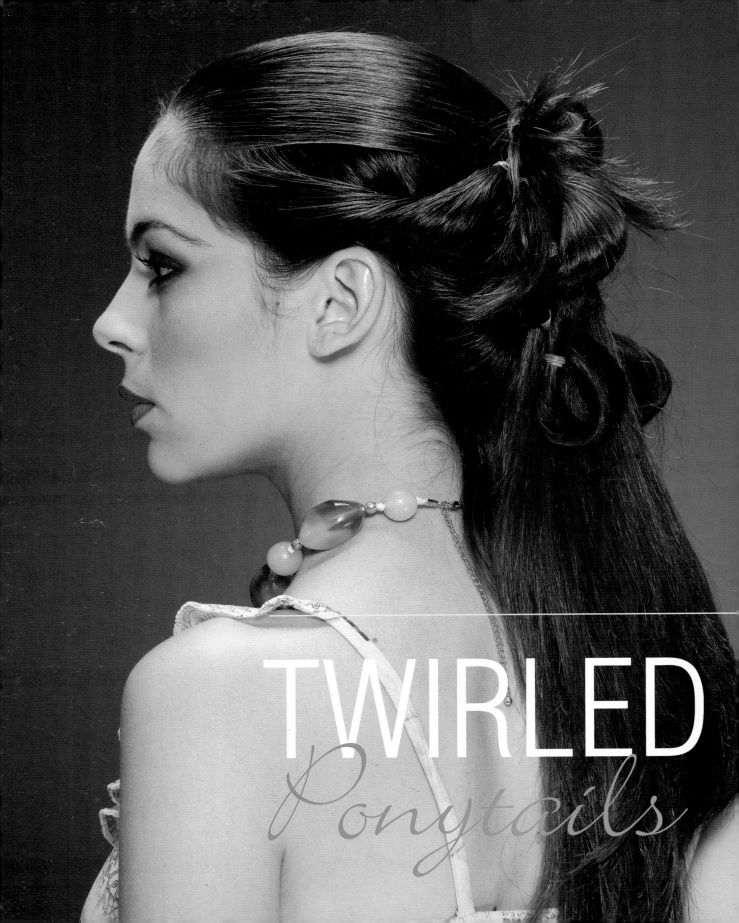

TWIRLED *Ponytails*

31

This is an excellent design for someone who isn't used to fussing with her hair. Just a few simple steps create an effect that is remarkable and distinct.

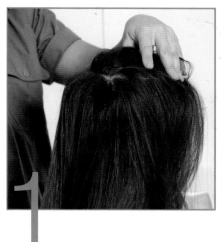

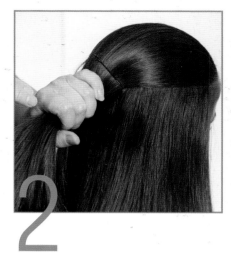

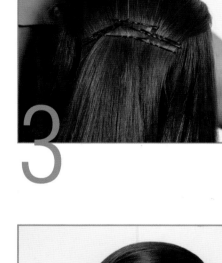

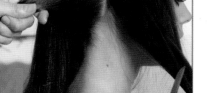

1. Wash and blow dry hair straight. Backcomb the hair at the crown to make a spongy base that is about 3 inches wide.

2. Brush the hair at the brow backwards, smoothing it over the spongy base.

3. Secure at the back of the head with a seam of pins.

4. Make a vertical part behind the right ear that extends from the spongy base to the neck.

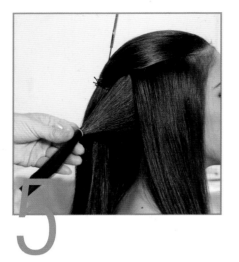

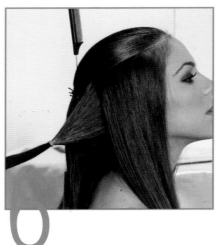

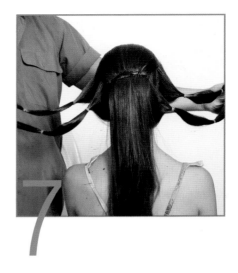

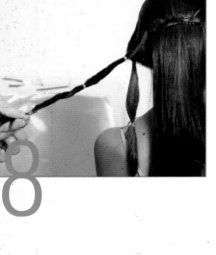

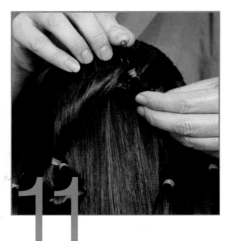

5. Gather the hair from a 1-inch section behind the part in a low ponytail, placing the elastic band far from the roots.

6. Place another elastic band on the same ponytail, about 4 inches below the first band.

7. Place another elastic band about 4 inches from the second one, near the end of the ponytail. Repeat to make a second ponytail just behind this one. Repeat to make similar ponytails on the other side of the head.

8. Grasp the ponytail on the left side of the head, closest to the spongy base, and twist it gently inwards.

9. Fold the ponytail upwards and towards the seam of pins at the top of the spongy base.

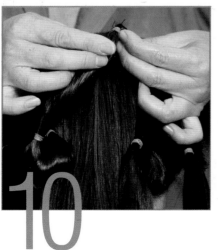

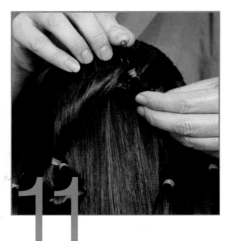

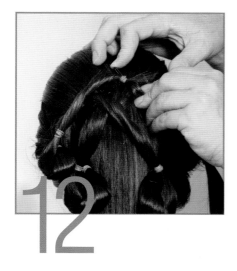

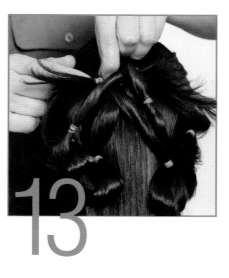

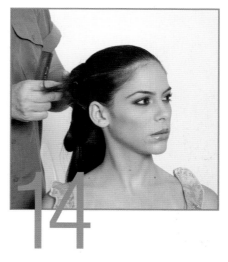

10. Insert a hairpin in the elastic band at the bottom of the ponytail.

11. Secure the ponytail to the spongy base.

12. Repeat on the right side of the head, twisting the ponytail closest to the spongy base and folding it upwards. Secure the ponytail with hairpins into the spongy base.

13. Move back to the left side and repeat with the second ponytail. Repeat with the second ponytail on the right side.

14. Mist with finishing spray.

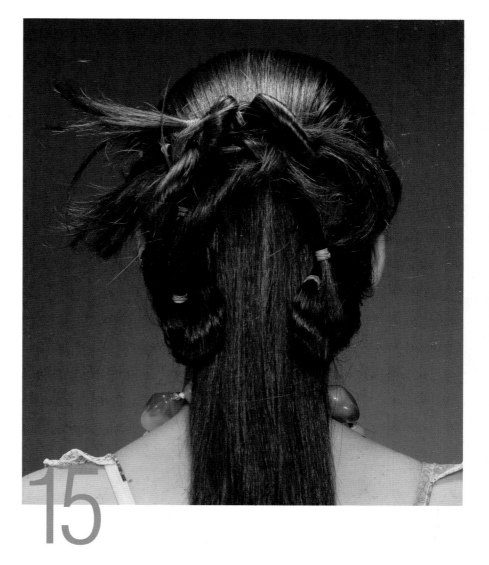

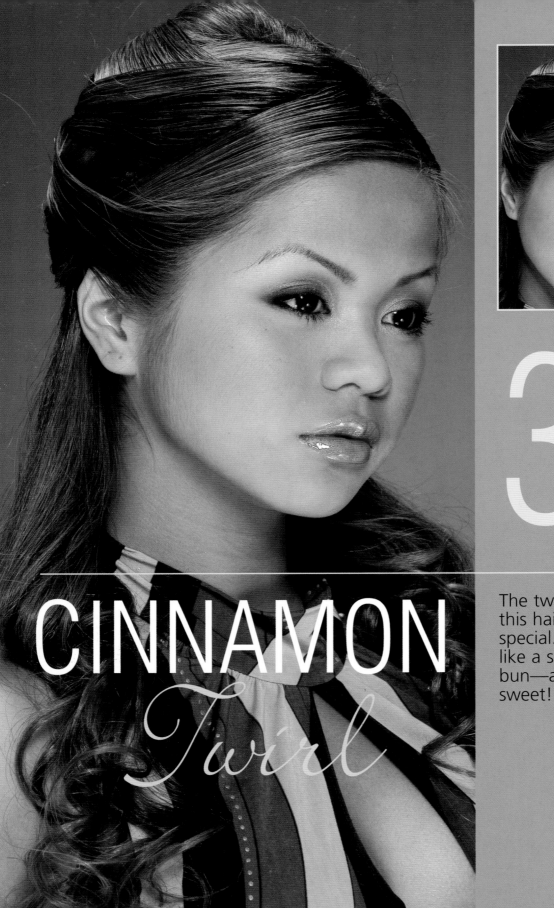

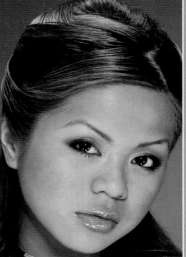

32

The twirl at the top of this hairstyle is really special. It looks a little like a spicy cinnamon bun—and is just as sweet!

CINNAMON
Twirl

1. Wash and blow dry hair wavy. Divide the hair into front and back sections with a part that extends from ear to ear over the crown. Make a left side part in the front hair. Backcomb the hair behind the part.

2. Lightly brush the hair at the crown over the backcombed section and secure with pins.

3. Brush the hair at the sides towards the back, securing with pins in a small half circle at the back of the head. Brush the hair into a flat strip and mist with holding spray.

4. Draw the strip of hair towards the right. Wrap the hair around a tail comb, then draw upwards.

5. Wrap the hair around another tail comb, then draw the hair towards the left. Draw the hair downwards then towards the right again, using tail combs for support, to wrap the hair into a buckle-style bun.

6. Divide the front hair with a zigzag part on the left side.

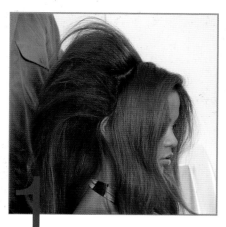

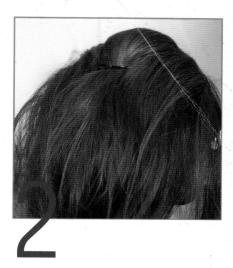

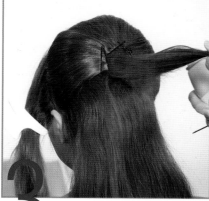

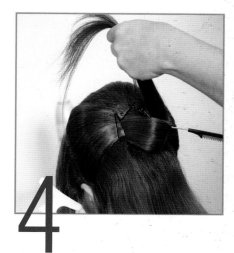

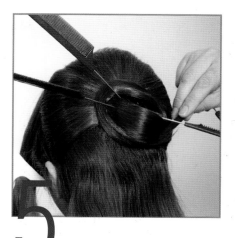

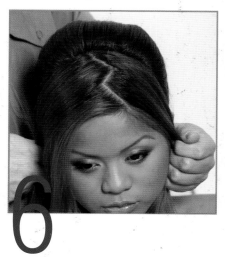

7. Grasp a section of hair from the right side of the part, just in front of the bun. Brush the hair into a flat strip and draw it backwards and towards the left. Wrap the hair around the bun and secure with a hairpin.

8. Grasp a section of hair from the front of the head, to the right of the first section. Brush the hair into a flat strip and draw it backwards over the cinnamon bun, making an X with the strip of hair in Step 7.

9. Repeat on the left side of the part, drawing two more sections of hair backwards to make an X of hair on the left side of the head. Grasp a section of hair from the left side of the part at the brow. Brush the hair into a flat strip and draw backwards.

10. Secure this section of hair under the bun with a hairpin.

11. Take a section of hair from the front right side of the part and draw backwards. Secure in the middle of the bun with a hairpin.

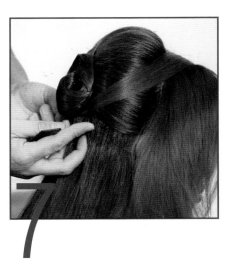

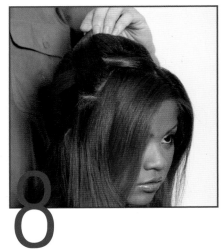

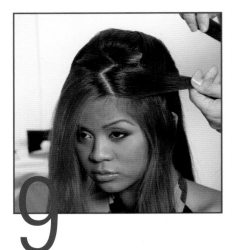

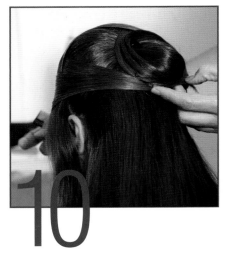

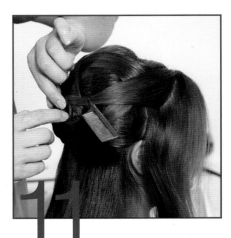

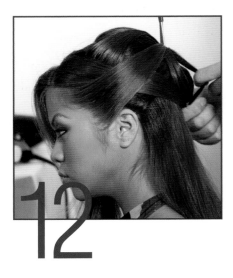

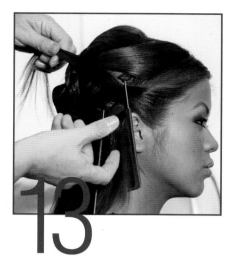

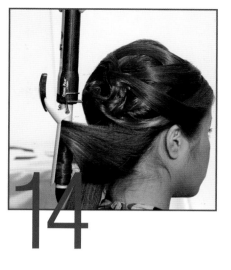

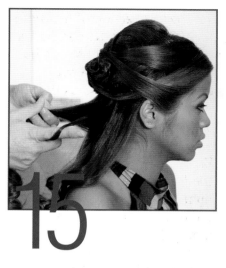

12. Take a section of hair from the front left side and draw downwards and backwards. Secure with a pin under the bun. Take another section of hair from this side of the head and draw upwards and backwards, making an X with the previous section. Draw this hair over the top of the bun and secure on the right side with hairpins.

13. Repeat on the left side of the head, drawing two sections of hair backwards to form an X of hair.

14. Curl the ends of the loose hair at the back of the head into ringlets with a curling iron.

15. Separate each ringlet into five sections.

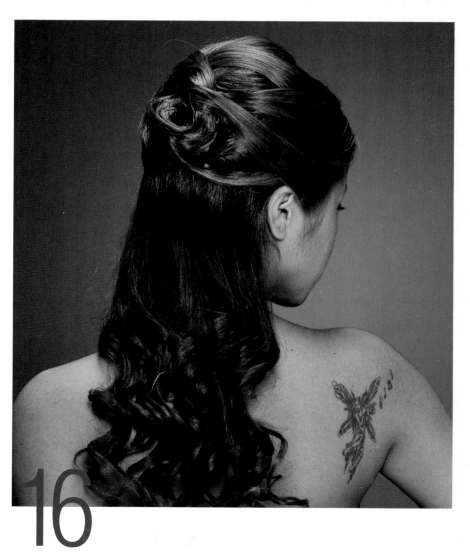

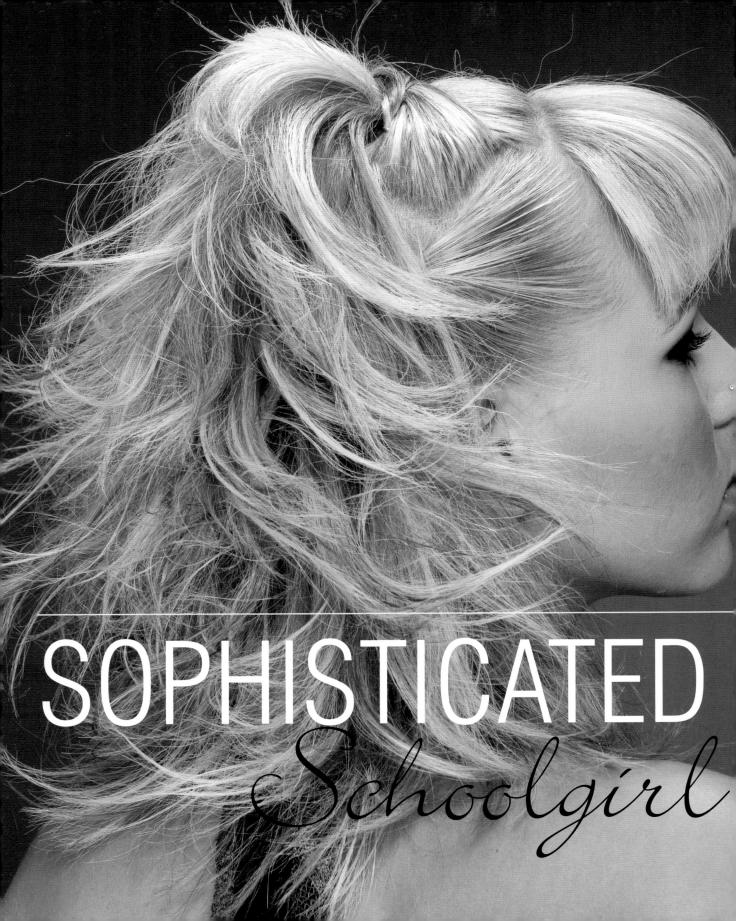

SOPHISTICATED
Schoolgirl

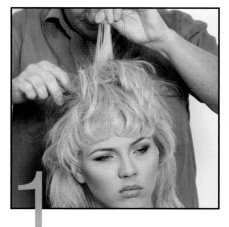

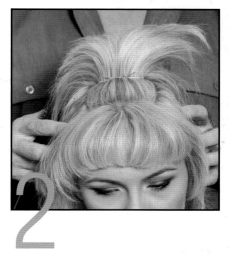

33

This youthful hairstyle is perfect for shoulder-length hair. It also gives added volume to hair that is naturally fine.

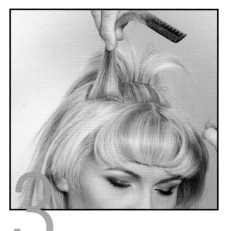

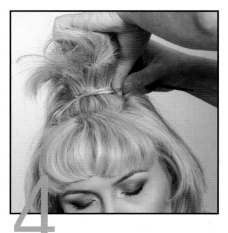

1. Wash and blow dry hair. Backcomb hair at the crown.

2. Brush the bangs forwards. Brush back the top hair at the crown and secure with a seam of pins that measures about 2 inches.

3. Make a triangular part to the right of the backcombed hair and brush the hair in this section upwards.

4. Twist the hair gently and secure on the left side of the seam of pins with a hairpin.

5. Make a triangular part on the left side of the head, just in front of the backcombed hair. Brush the hair in this section upwards.

6. Twist the hair gently and secure on the right side of the seam of pins with a hairpin.

7. Make triangular parts on the right and left side of the back-combed section. These parts should be in a straight line with the parts you made in Steps 3 and 5. Brush the hair in these sections upwards and hold with a clip on top of the head.

8. Brush the hair at the front right side of the head backwards and twist upwards.

9. Pin the hair at the back of the head, just below the hair being held at the top with a clip. Repeat on the left side of the head. Remove the clip from the top of the head, letting hair fall over the twisted sections.

10. Brush the loose hair at the back of the head upwards and mist with finishing spray.

11. Blow dry hair upwards to create a naturally thick look.

12. Let the hair fall loose and spray again with finishing spray.

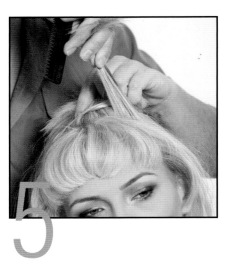
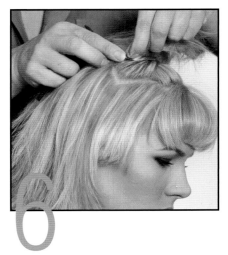
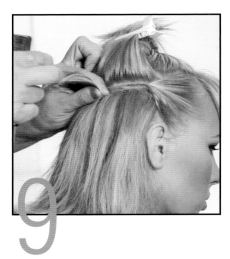
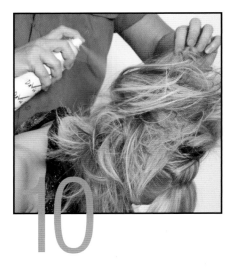
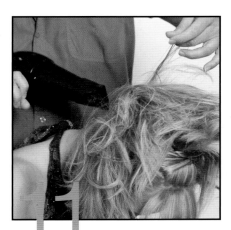
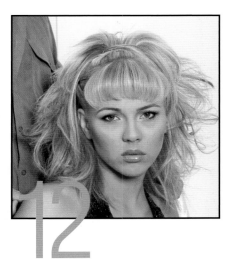

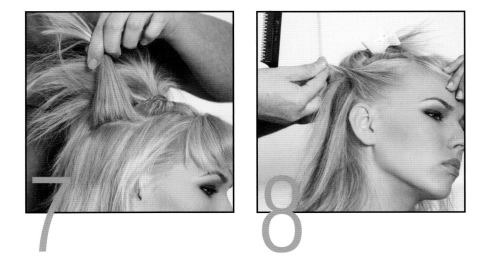

7

8

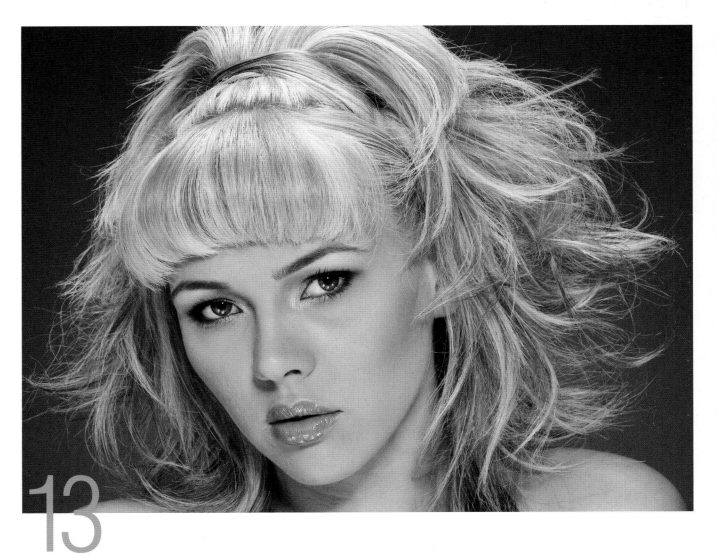

13

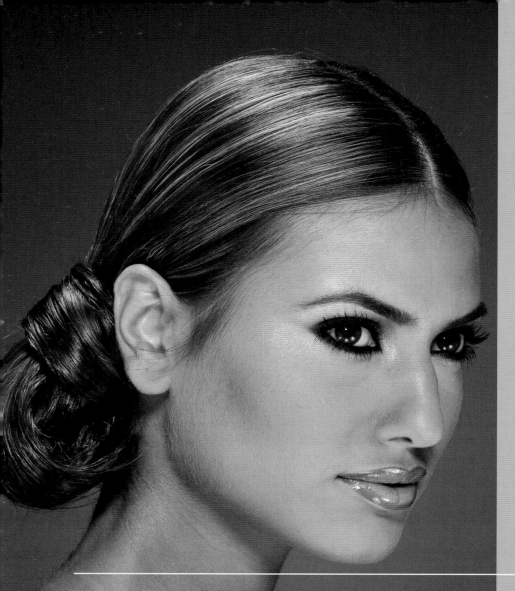

34

BEADED
Brilliance

A simple hairstyle accented with a striking accessory creates an effect that is no less than brilliant. This is a great design for showing off a special hair accessory.

1. Wash and blow dry hair straight.

2. Divide the hair into left and right sections by making a middle part from the brow to the nape of the neck. Gather the hair in each section in a low ponytail behind each ear.

3. Start with the ponytail on the right, backcombing it to add volume.

4. Gently comb the hair to make a flat strip.

5. Fold the ponytail inwards towards the nape of the neck.

6. Secure with bobby pins at the hairline, leaving the ends loose.

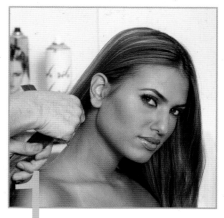

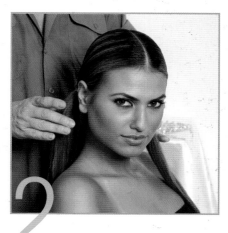

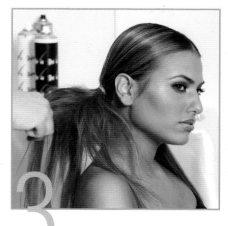

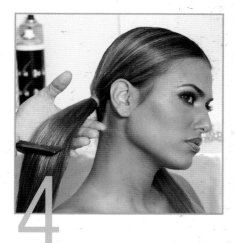

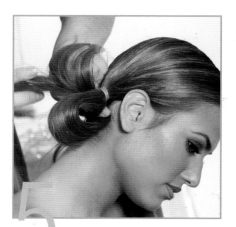

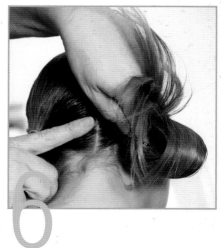

7. Brush the loose ends upwards on the left side of the ponytail.

8. Wrap the ends of the ponytail over the elastic band to conceal it and draw downwards on the right side of the ponytail.

9. Secure the ends with bobby pins.

10. Repeat with the ponytail on the left side, brushing it into a flat strip and folding it inwards towards the nape of the neck.

11. Gently spread out the hair in the ponytails to form upside-down fans. Spray both ponytails with finishing spray.

12. You can add a beaded hair accessory to complete the look.

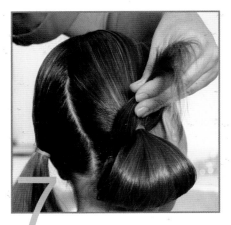

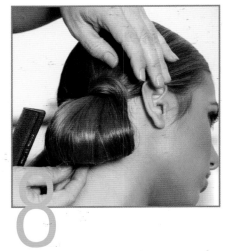

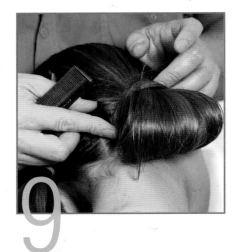

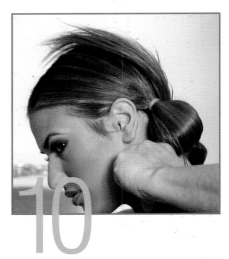

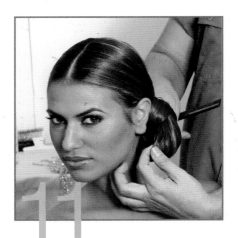

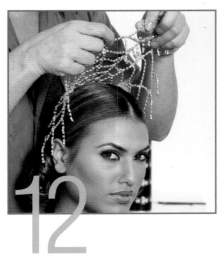

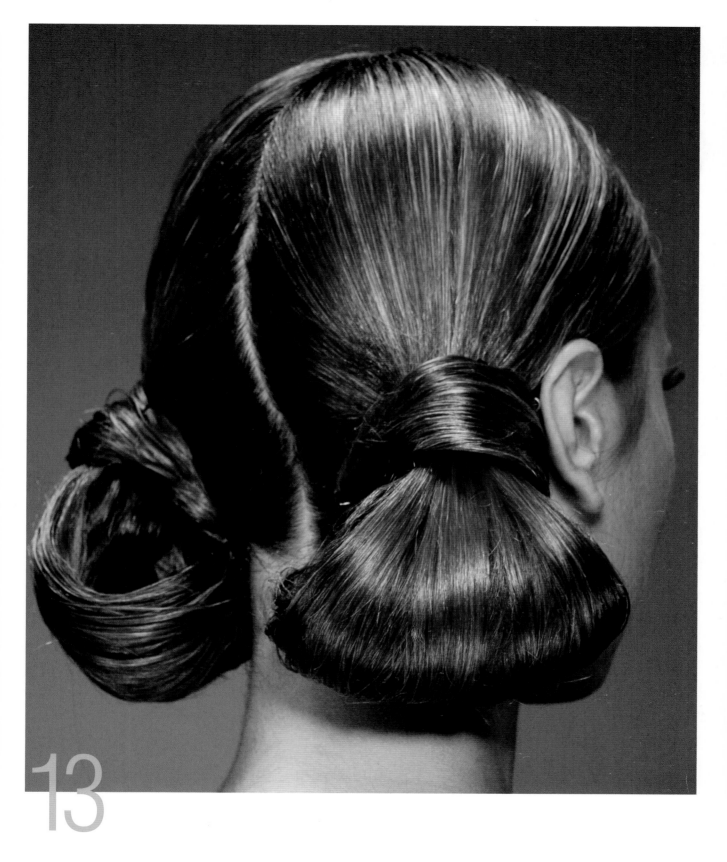

13

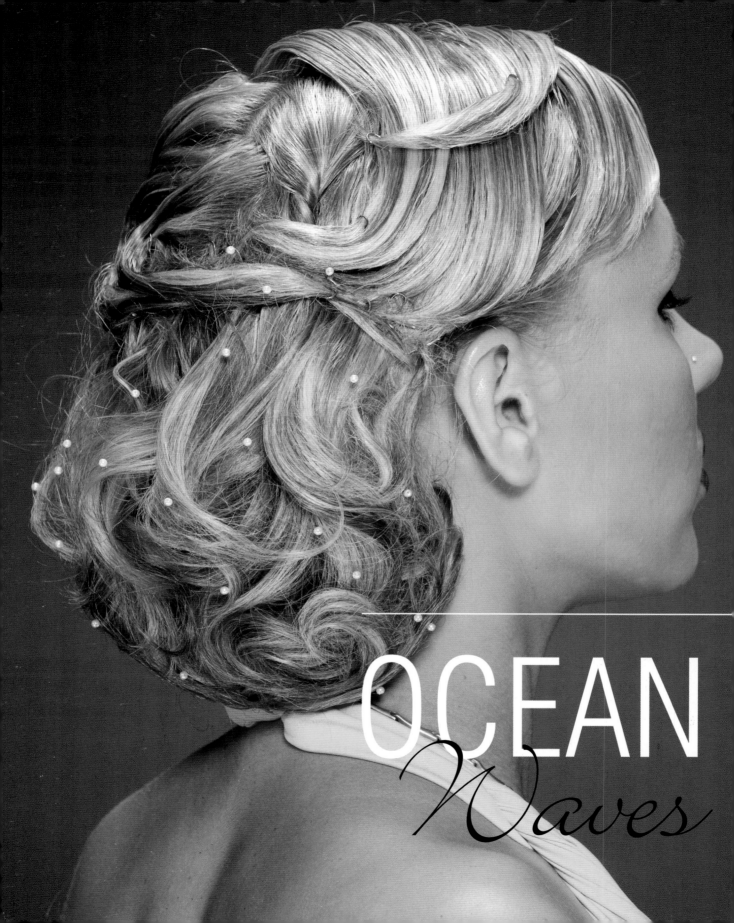

OCEAN

Waves

35

Locks of hair flow gently from the front to the back in a natural motion that recalls rolling waves.

1. Massage strong styling mousse into the hair and set in rollers.

2. Remove the rollers and brush out the hair. Make side parts on the right and left sides of the head that extend from the brow to the middle of the head.

3. Brush the hair on the right side of the part downwards and secure with a seam of pins behind the right ear. Repeat on the left side of the head, and secure the hair behind the left ear. Leave a rectangular section of hair at the top of the head loose.

4. Take a lock of hair from the middle section and twist it outwards. Draw the hair backwards and secure near the seam of pins behind the right ear.

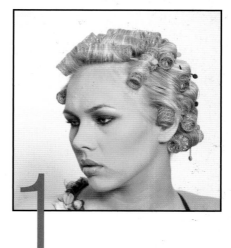

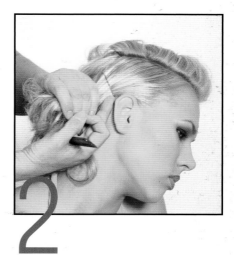

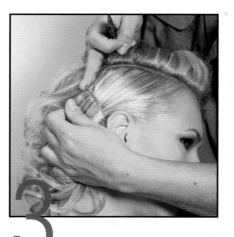

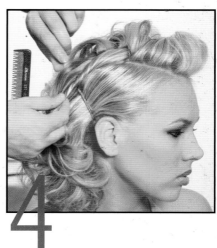

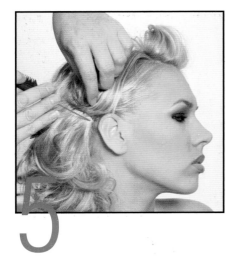

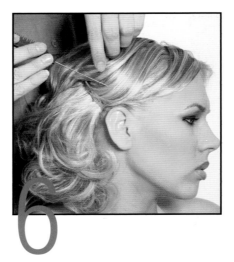

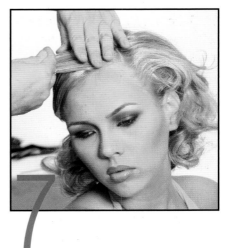

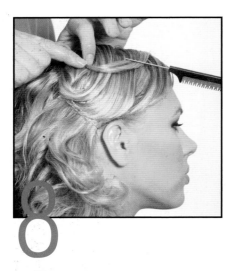

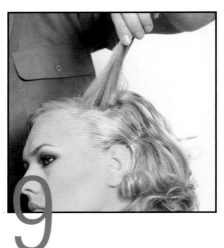

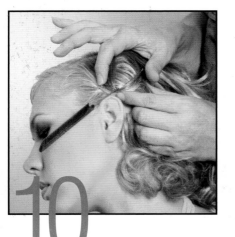

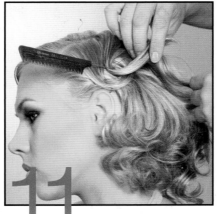

5. Take another lock of hair from the middle section and draw it downwards, towards the right ear. Draw the hair over the seam of pins to conceal it. Curve the hair in an arc upwards, and secure with pins.

6. Take another lock of hair, this one closer to the front of the head. Draw the hair over the seam of pins to conceal it, and curve in an arc towards the back. Secure with bobby pins.

7. Take a lock of hair from the left side of the middle section. Draw it over the middle section, towards the right side of the head.

8. Curve the hair into an arc towards the back of the head, using a tail comb for support. Secure this lock above the other locks.

9. Take a lock of hair from the left side of the middle section. Brush the lock downwards, towards the seam of pins on the left side of the head.

10. Use a tail comb for support and curve the hair into an arc over the seam of pins. Secure with a bobby pin.

11. Take another lock of hair from the middle section and curve in an arc on the left side of the head, close to the previous one.

12. Take another lock of hair behind this one and curve into an arc to cover the pins in the previous arc.

13. Repeat to make a series of arcs on the left side of the head, continuing until you reach the locks from the right side of the head.

14. Mist the hair with holding spray and blow dry.

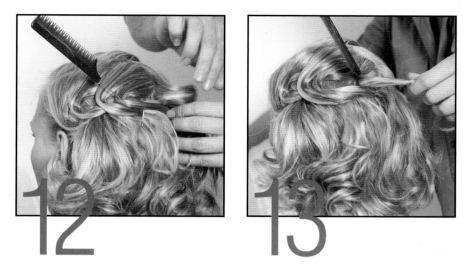

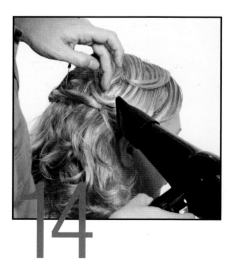

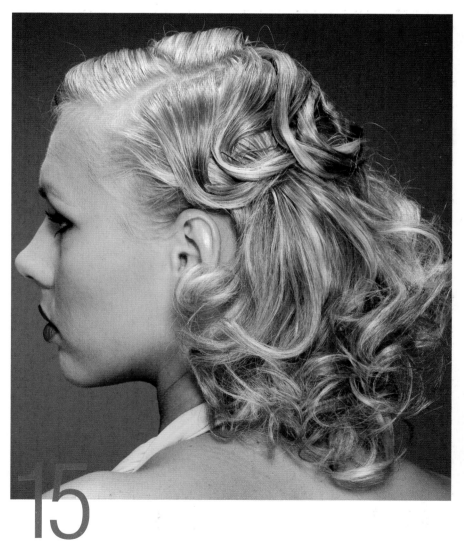

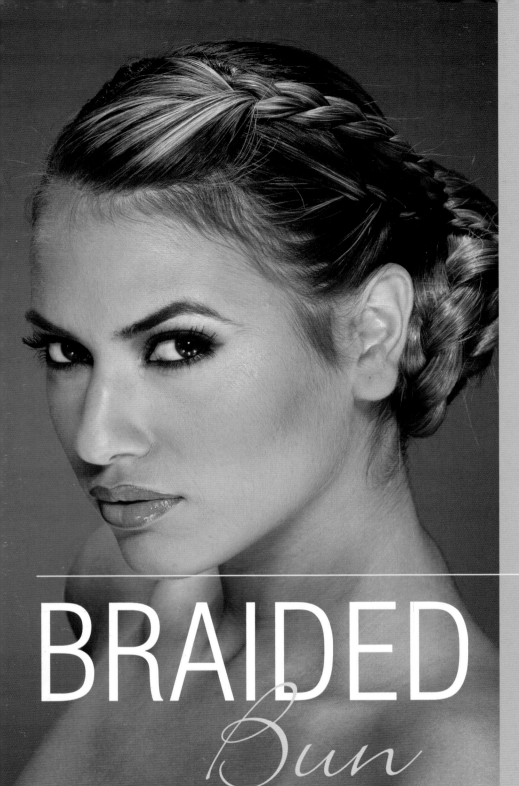

BRAIDED
Bun

36

Add volume to long hair with the hair extension in this design. Though the final look is intricate, the steps are deceptively simple.

1. Wash and blow dry hair straight. Divide the hair into front and back sections with a part that extends from the top of each ear over the crown. Make a right side part in the front hair. Gather the back hair in a low ponytail. Select a long hair extension.

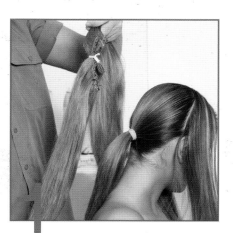

2. Sew the extension using a blunt needle and thick thread above the natural ponytail. Divide the extension into right and left sections and draw the natural ponytail upwards between the two sections.

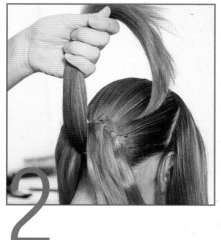

3. Brush the ponytail upwards.

4. Roll the ponytail inwards over a finger.

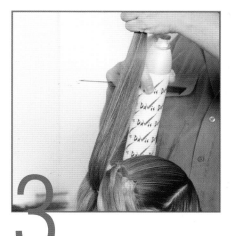

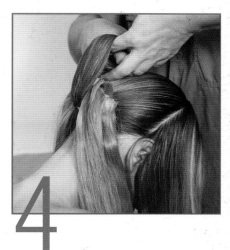

5. Secure the rolled ponytail to the head with bobby pins at either side, making a right-side-up fan that conceals the stitches securing the extension.

6. Plait the extension hair on either side of the ponytail into braids.

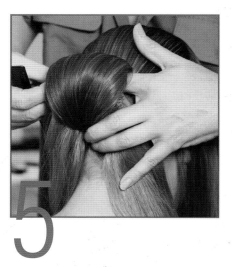

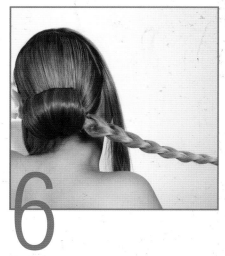

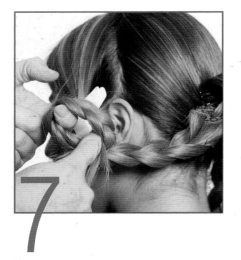

7

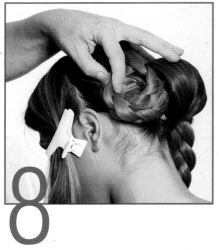

8

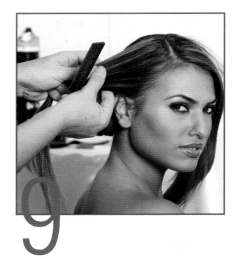

9

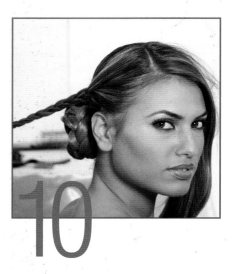

10

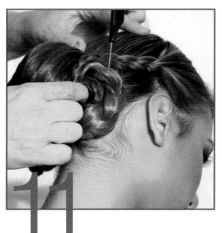

11

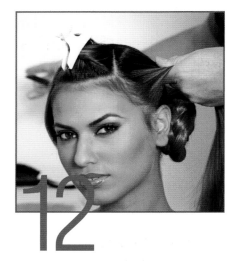

12

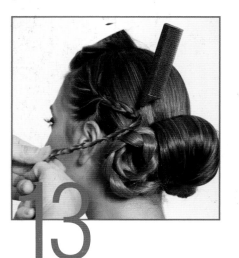

13

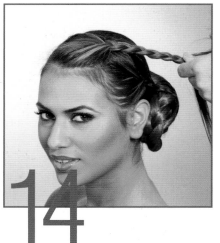

14

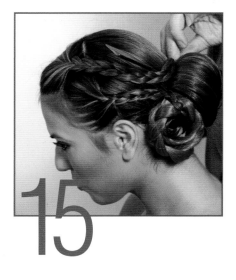

15

7. Coil the braid on the left side upwards and inwards to form a braided spiral.

8. Place the braided spiral over the opening on the left side of the fan and secure with hairpins. Repeat on the right side of the head, coiling the braid into a braided spiral and securing with hairpins.

9. Brush back the hair on the right of the part.

10. Plait the hair into a braid.

11. Draw the braid to the back of the head and coil to form a braided spiral. Secure near the coiled braid extension.

12. Move to the hair on the left side of the part. Hold the bangs in a clip. Brush back the hair to the left of the bangs and plait into a braid.

13. Draw the braid towards the back of the head and coil to form a braided spiral. Secure with pins to the coiled braid extension.

14. Plait a braid with the bangs.

15. Draw the braid backwards and secure with pins at the top of the right-side-up fan.

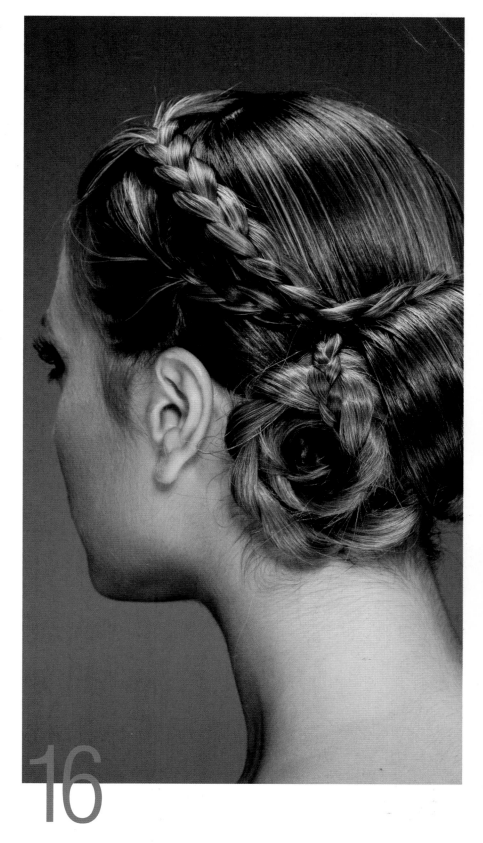

16

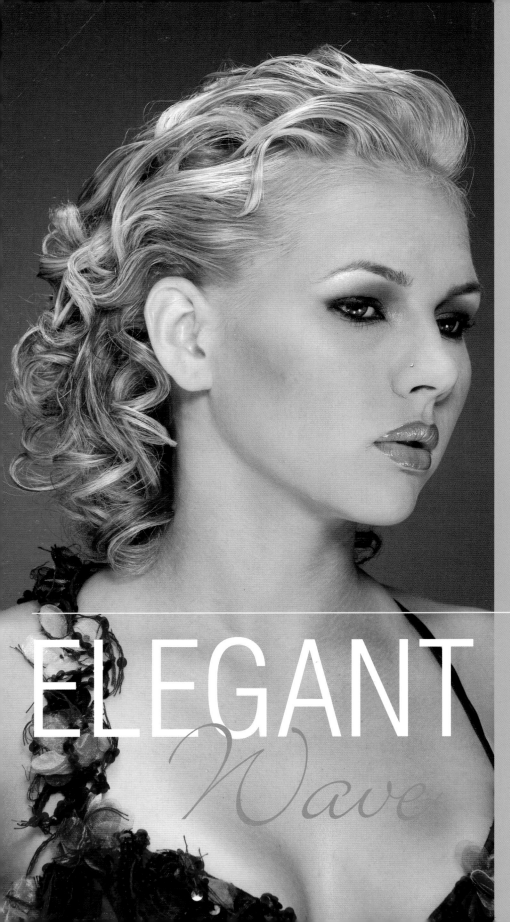

37

ELEGANT *Wave*

The curls in this design are tucked into each other carefully and gracefully, creating a subtly sculpted look.

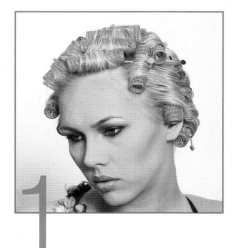

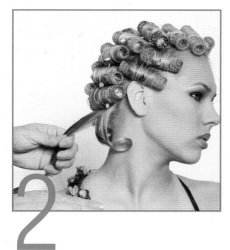

1. Wash hair and set in hot rollers.

2. After the hair cools, release each roller separately, starting at the nape of the neck. Separate each roll into three or four locks of hair.

3. Continue releasing the hair from the rollers, working your way up the back of the head, and separating each roll into several locks of hair.

4. Continue in this manner until the middle of the head. Divide each roll of hair in this area into four locks.

5. From the middle of the head and until the bangs, divide each roll of hair into two locks.

6. Weave each lock of hair at the back of the head between two locks of hair by tucking the upper lock between the lower locks.

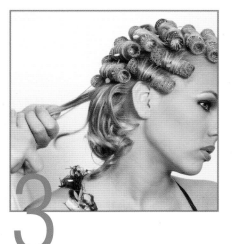

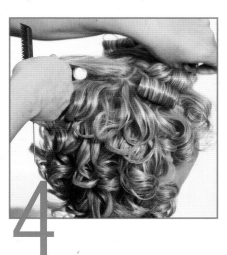

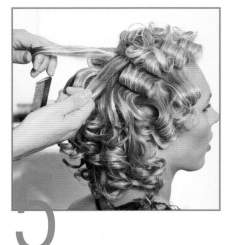

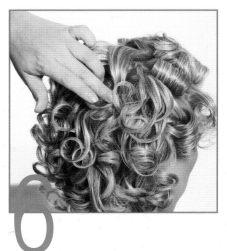

7. Secure the upper locks with hairpins.

8. Repeat the same action, this time tucking locks of hair at the sides of the head between locks of hair that are lower down.

9. Use hairpins to secure the upper locks.

10. Continue in this manner, working your way to the front of the head, releasing the rollers and dividing the hair into two locks.

11. Then tuck the locks of hair between lower locks of hair.

12. Arrange the curls so that they are tidy yet carefree.

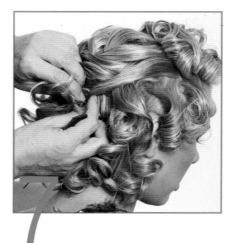

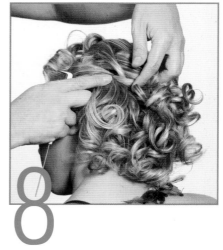

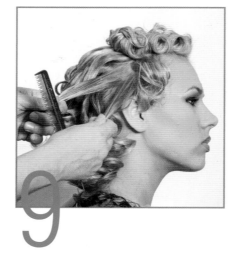

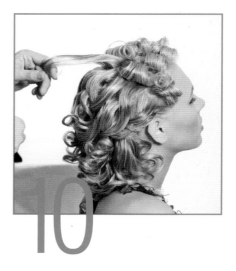

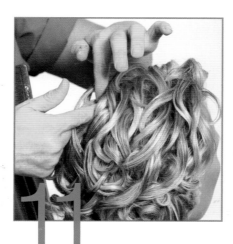

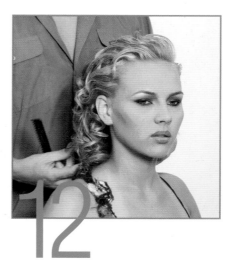

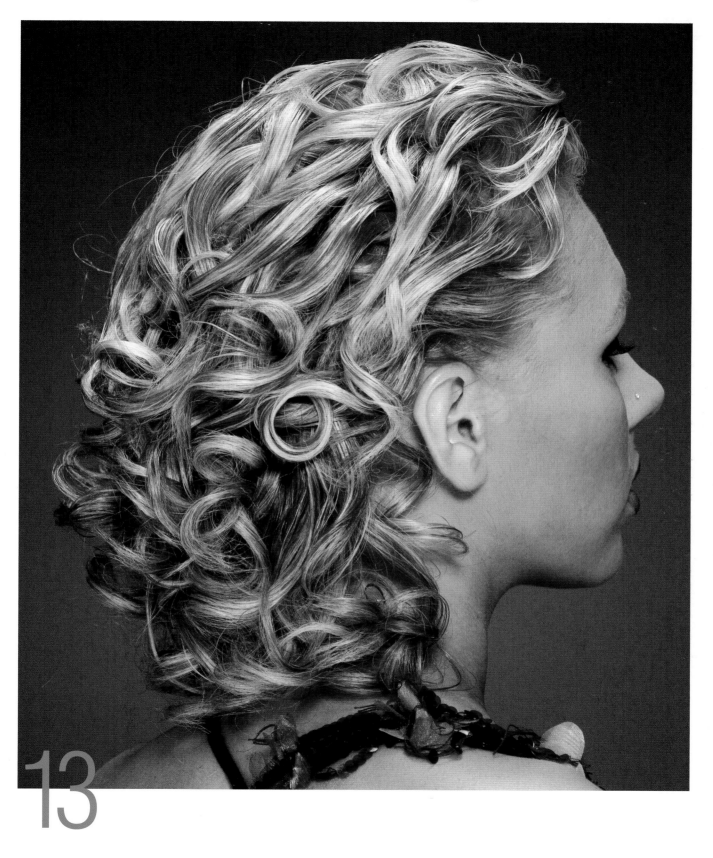

13

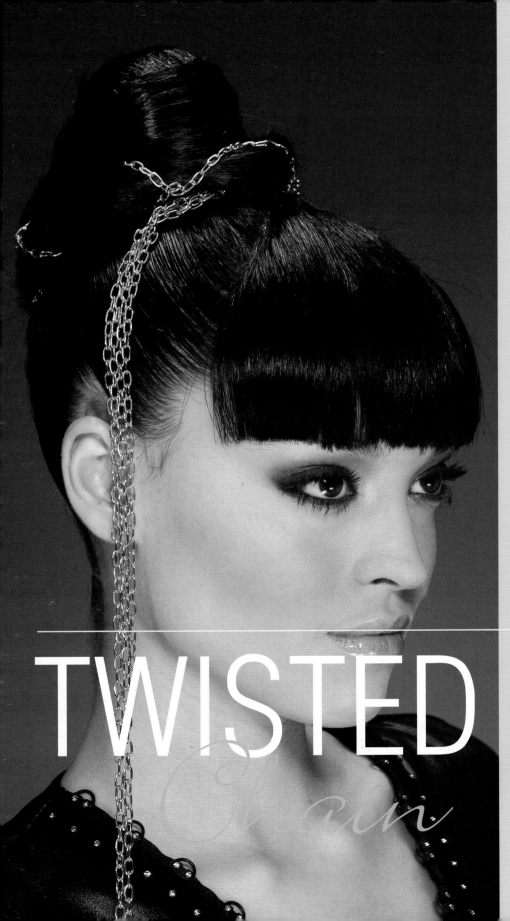

38

TWISTED

Chain

Maximize the sleekness of this style by ensuring the front hair is smoothly drawn backwards. Integrating a chain adds a surprising dazzle.

1. Wash and blow dry hair straight. Hold the bangs with a clip and gather the rest of the hair in a ponytail at the crown. Select a long hair extension.

2. Divide the extension into right and left sections.

3. Lay the extension on the top of the ponytail so that one section hangs on either side of the ponytail.

4. Draw the two sections of the extension to the back of the ponytail and join in a ponytail.

5. Mist the natural ponytail with holding spray.

6. Brush the natural ponytail forwards and fold, making a small mound on the top of the head.

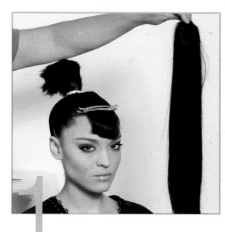

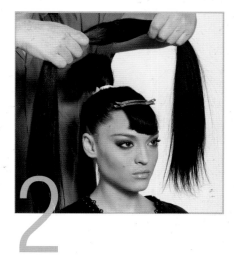

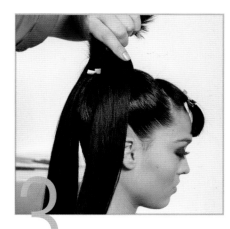

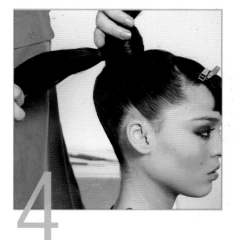

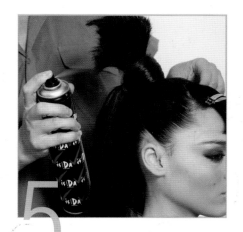

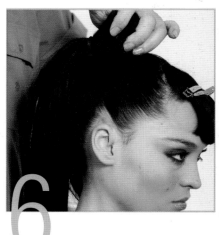

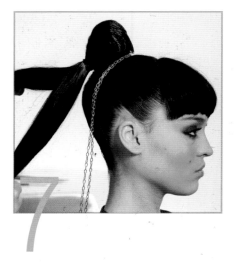

7

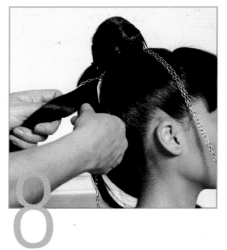

8

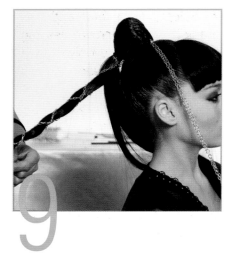

9

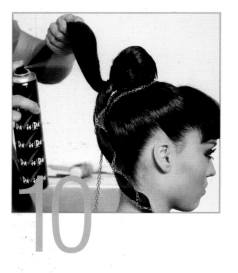

10

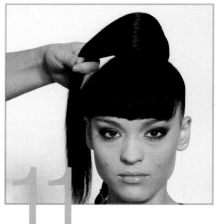

11

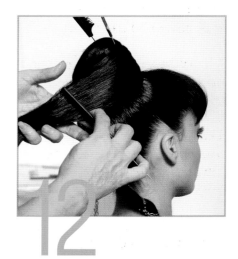

12

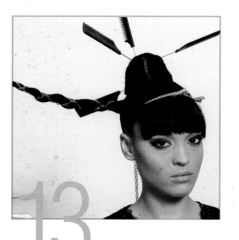

13

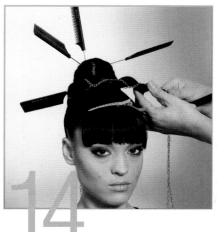

14

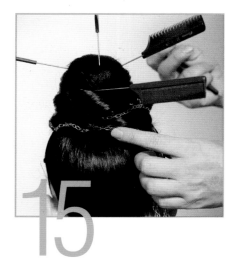

15

7. Select a long chain and drape it over the crown, leaving the ends to hang evenly on either side of the head.

8. Divide the extension into right and left sections. Plait the right section with two sides of the chain to make a braid.

9. Continue braiding the chain and extension to make a long chain braid.

10. Brush the left section of the extension into a wide strip and mist with holding spray.

11. Wrap the strip around the front of the mound on top of the head.

12. Draw the strip towards the back, so that it forms a cone at the top of the head. Support the cone with tail combs.

13. Lift the chain braid at the back of the head upwards.

14. Wrap the braid around the base of the cone.

15. Draw the braid towards the back of the head and secure with hairpins. Use hairpins to secure the cone, then mist with finishing spray.

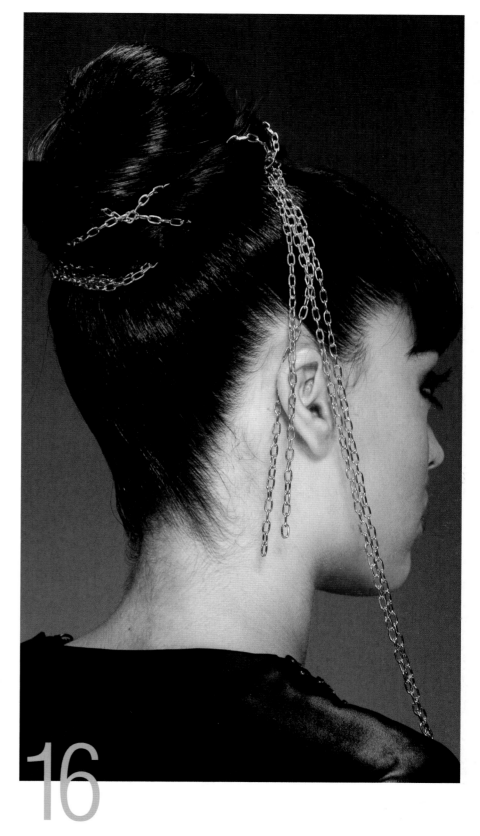

16

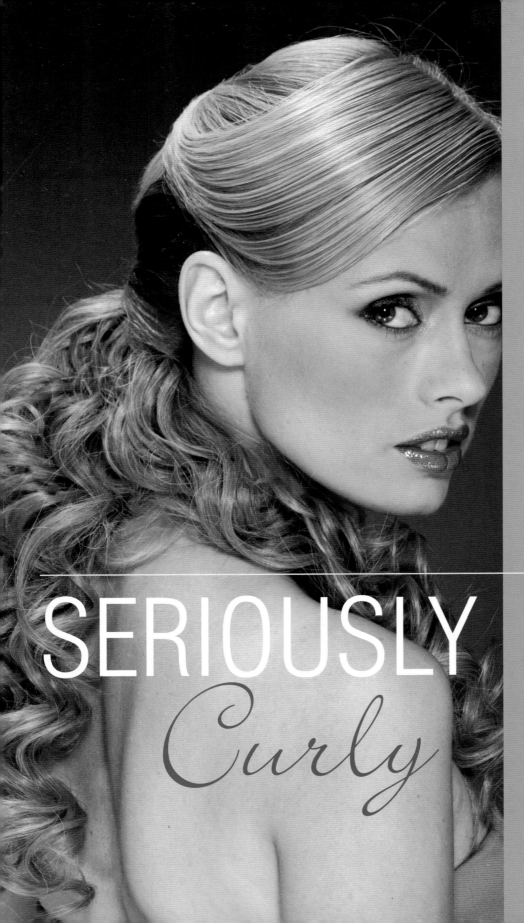

39

SERIOUSLY
Curly

Add length and volume to your look with the curly hair extension in this design. The front of the style is seriously straight; the back is curiously curly.

1. Wash and blow dry hair wavy. Make a rectangular part from the crown to the nape of the neck that is 4 inches wide. Brush the hair in this section downwards. Hold the hair to the right and left in clips.

2. Backcomb the hair at the top of the rectangle to make a spongy base.

3. Mist with holding spray and blow dry on medium heat.

4. Select a long hair extension and curl into ringlets with a curling iron.

5. Sew the extension to the spongy base using a blunt needle and thick thread.

6. Make a diagonal part above the extension, on the right side. Gather the hair in this section and draw diagonally downwards while twisting.

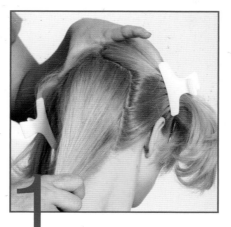

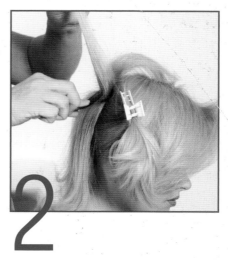

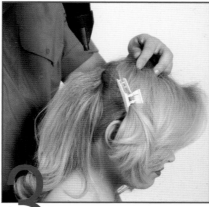

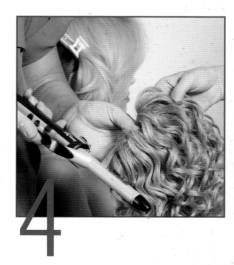

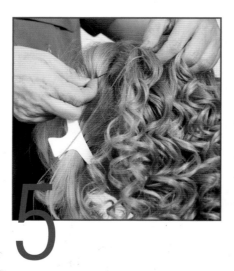

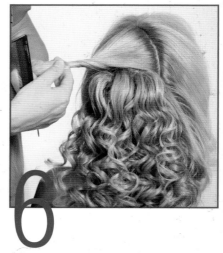

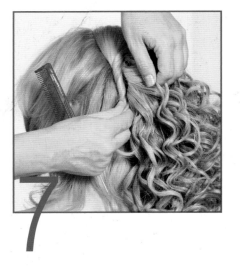

7

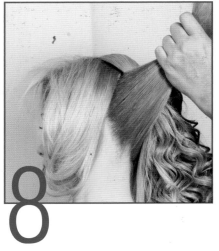

8

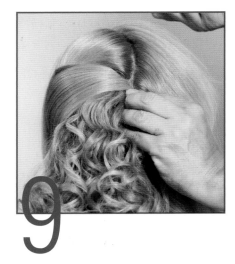

9

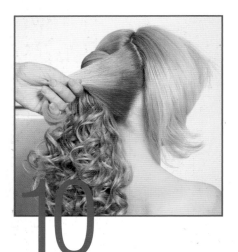

10

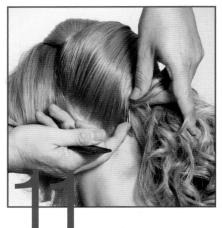

11

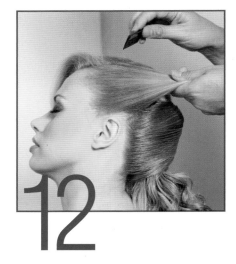

12

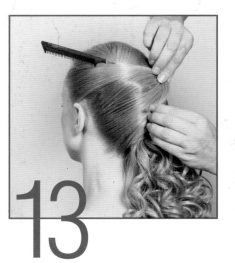

13

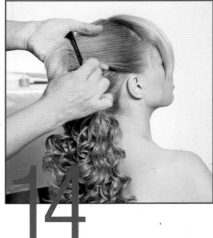

14

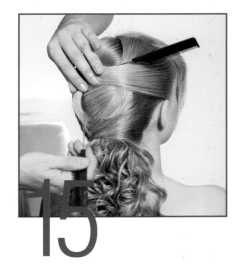

15

7. Tuck the hair on the left side of the extension and secure with hairpins.

8. Gather the hair on the left side of the head, from the ear to the nape of the neck. Brush the hair upwards and draw over to the right side.

9. Twist the hair gently upwards and secure with pins on the right side of the extension.

10. Gather a similar section of hair on the right side, from the ear to the nape of the neck. Brush the hair upwards and draw over to the left side.

11. Twist the hair gently upwards and secure with pins on the left side of the head, under the section drawn over in Step 8.

12. Brush the front hair on the left side backwards.

13. Mist the hair with holding spray and draw into a wave-like shape at the back of the head on the right side. Use a tail comb for support, then secure with hairpins.

14. Repeat on the other side of the head, brushing the hair backwards.

15. Mist the hair with holding spray and draw into a wave-like shape. Use a tail comb for support, then secure with a hairpin.

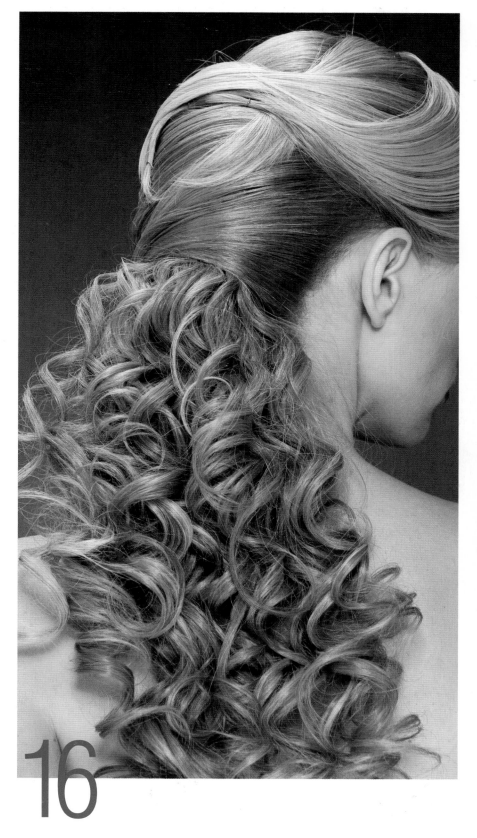

16

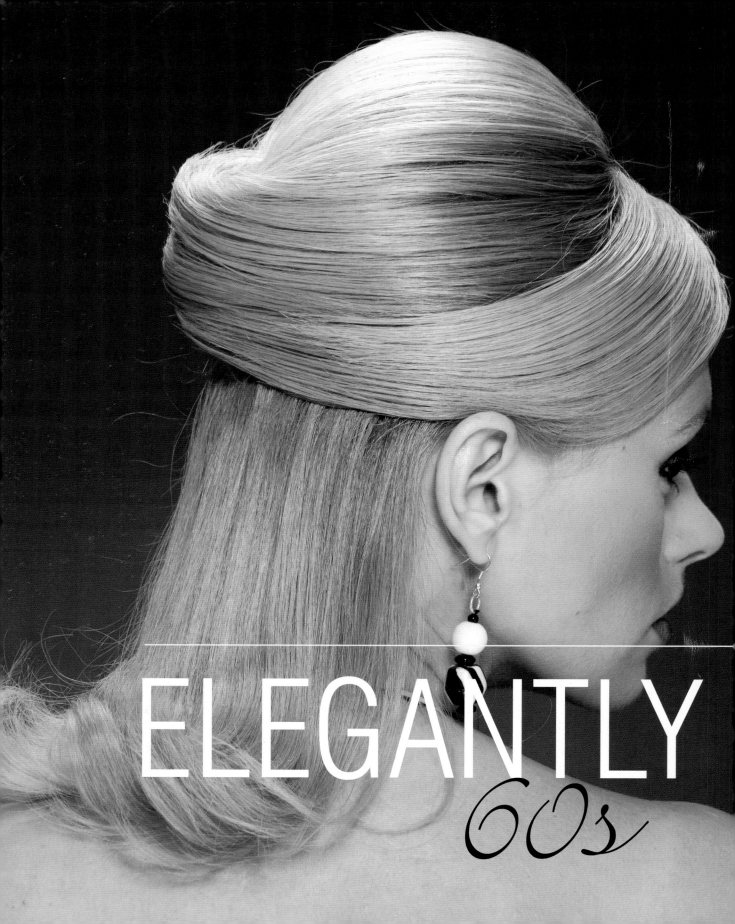

ELEGANTLY

60s

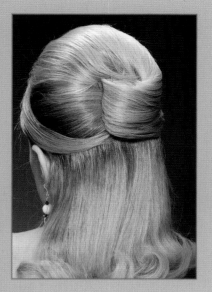

40

Elegance is always in style. Even though this design is inspired by the great beauties of the 1960s, it remains perfectly fashionable today.

1. Wash and blow dry hair, brushing it with a round brush to make outward curls at the ends. Divide the hair into front and back sections with a part that extends from ear to ear over the crown. Backcomb the hair just behind the part.

2. Backcomb all of the hair along the part.

3. Gently brush the front hair over the backcombed section to add volume at the top.

4. Brush the hair on the left side towards the back of the head and secure with a seam of bobby pins.

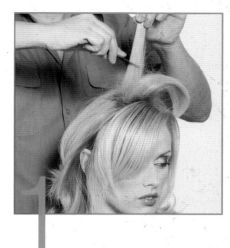

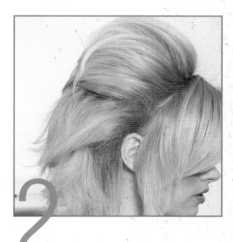

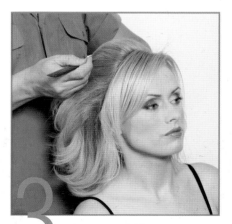

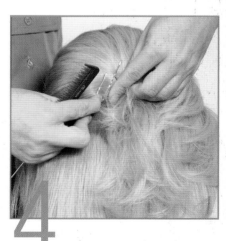

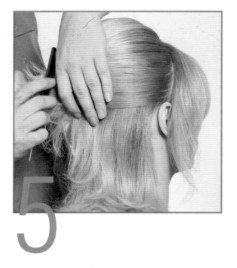

5

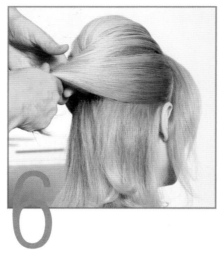

6

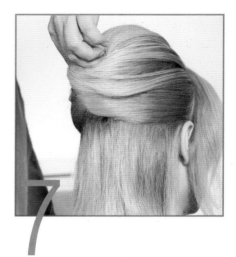

7

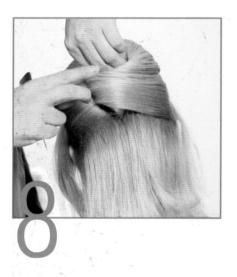

8

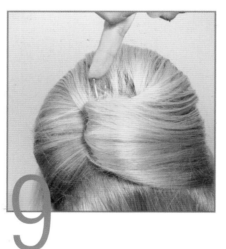

9

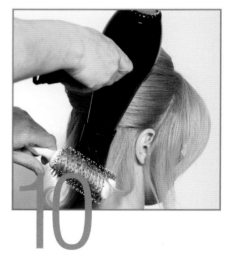

10

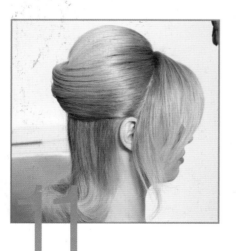

11

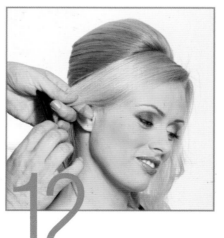

12

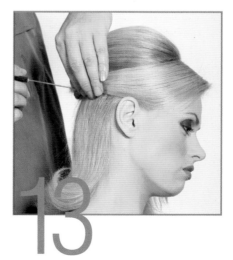

13

5. Brush the hair on the right side towards the back of the head.

6. Twist the hair upwards around a finger.

7. Draw the ends of the hair upwards.

8. Tuck the hair inwards to form an upright twist.

9. Secure the twist with hairpins and mist with holding spray.

10. Blow dry the loose hair at the back of the head, using a round brush to make outwards curls at the ends.

11. Make a right side part in the front hair.

12. Brush the hair on the right side of the part downwards and backwards.

13. Draw the hair around the bottom of the upright twist so that it curves naturally. Secure with hairpins at the back of the head.

14. Brush the hair on the left side downwards and backwards, and draw around the bottom of the upright twist, securing with pins at the back of the head.

15. Mist with holding spray to create a smooth, sleek finish.

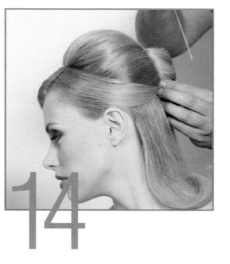

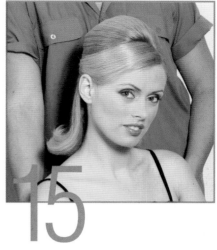

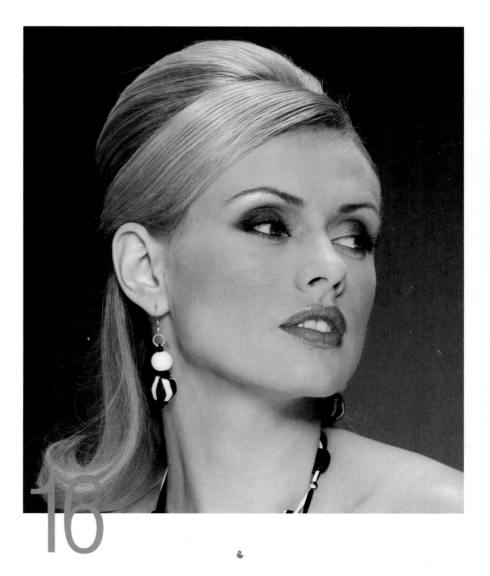

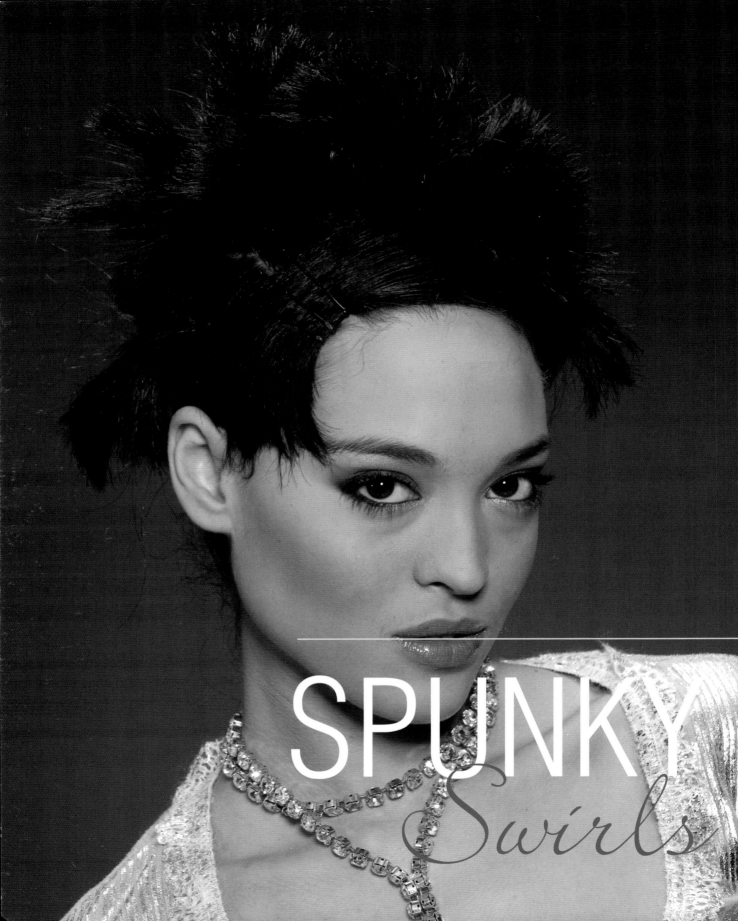

SPUNKY
Swirls

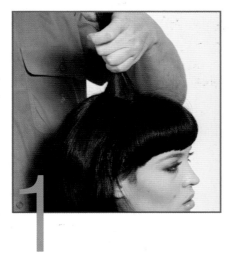

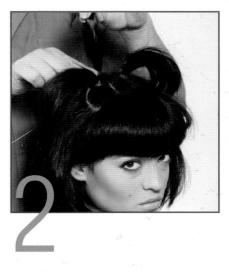

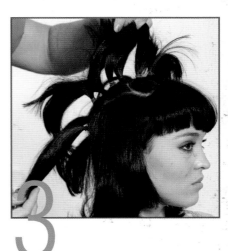

1. Wash and blow dry hair straight. Make a ponytail with a 1-inch section of hair at the crown.

2. Make a similar ponytail to the right of the first ponytail.

3. Make a ponytail behind these ponytails that is similar in size. Continue making ponytails down the middle of the head.

4. Make similar ponytails all over the head, leaving the bangs loose.

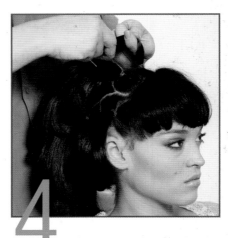

41

Looking for an easy way to add spunk to your life? Try wearing these swirled ponytails. They are easy to make, and fun to wear.

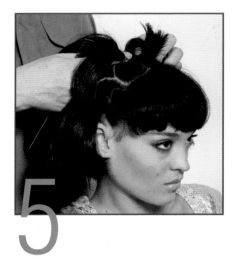

5

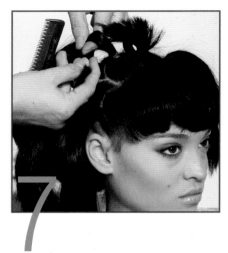

6

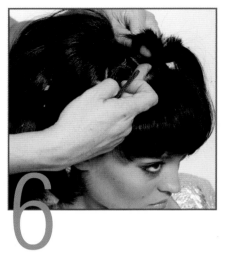

7

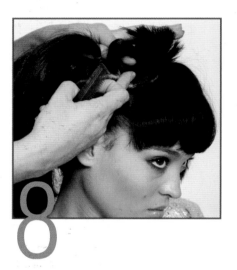

8

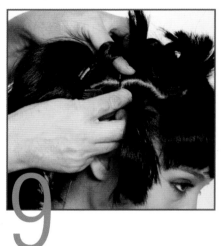

9

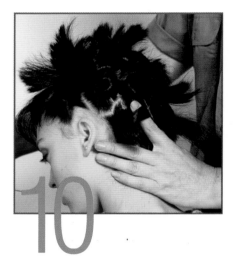

10

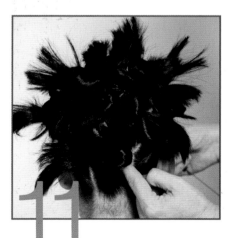

11

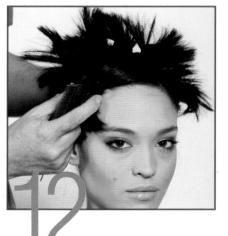

12

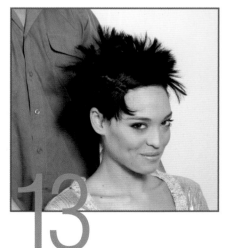

13

5. Start with a ponytail at the top of the head. Roll one ponytail over a finger to make a loop.

6. Secure the loop with a bobby pin, leaving the ends loose.

7. Roll another ponytail over a finger into a loop.

8. Secure the loop with a bobby pin, leaving the ends loose.

9. Continue to roll ponytails and pin them in this manner.

10. Work your way from the top of the head to the nape of the neck.

11. Mist hair with holding spray to secure the loops.

12. Brush the bangs to the right and secure with bobby pins, drawing the ends along the face.

13. Mist with holding spray.

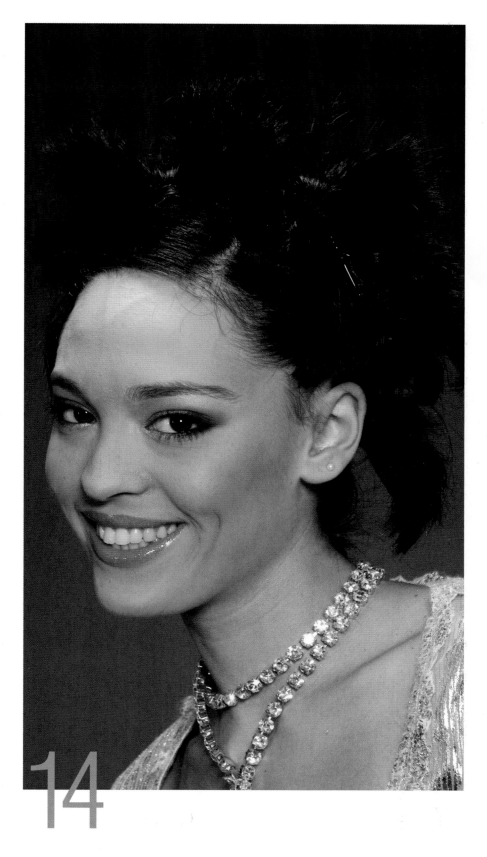

14

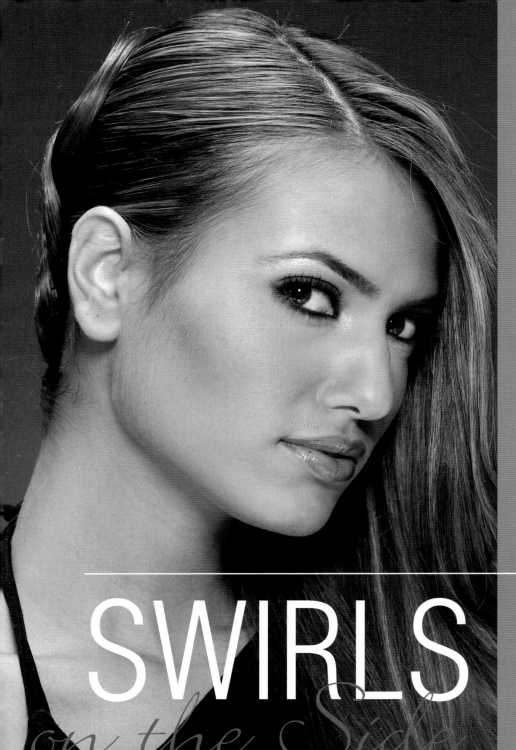

42

SWIRLS
on the Side

Create two looks with one style. The right side is delicately swirled; the left side hangs loose and untamed. The effect is unexpected and distinct.

1. Wash and blow dry hair straight. Make a right side part from the brow to behind the right ear. Gather the hair in front of the part in a clip. Backcomb the hair behind the part, starting at the top of the head.

2. Backcomb the hair behind the part to the nape of the neck, making a spongy base along the part.

3. Brush the hair on the right side of the head backwards.

4. Draw the hair upwards so that it conceals the spongy base.

5. Secure the hair with a seam of pins that runs along the spongy base.

6. Draw a lock of hair from the top of the seam of pins. Mist with holding spray and draw downwards, then forwards. Use a tail comb for support.

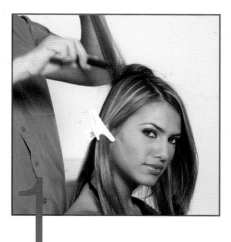

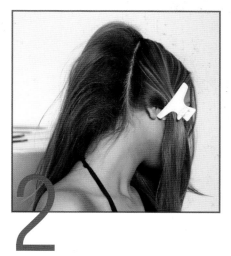

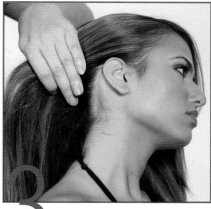

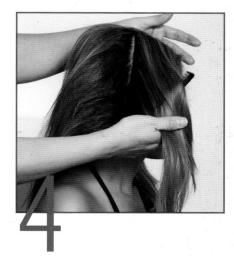

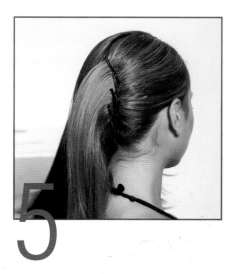

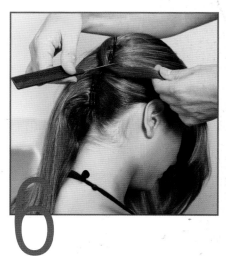

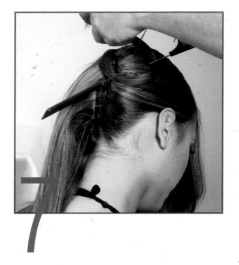

7

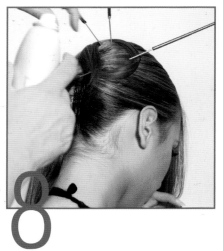

8

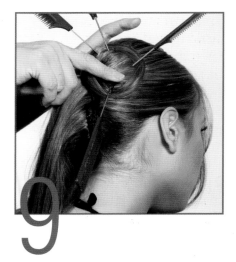

9

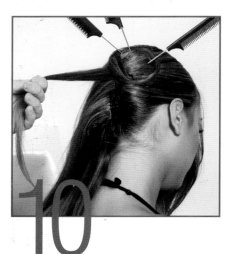

10

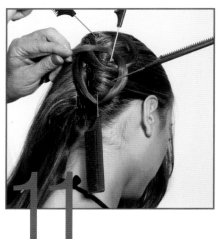

11

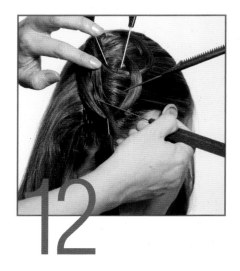

12

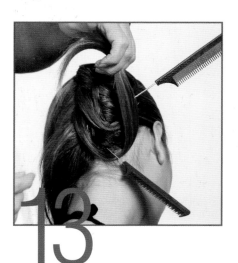

13

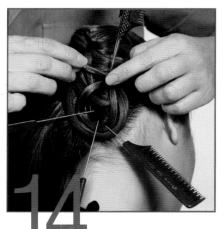

14

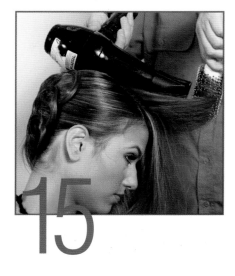

15

7. Now draw the lock of hair upwards and backwards, using a tail comb for support, to form a large U shape.

8. Draw the hair over the top of the head and backwards, towards the seam of pins.

9. Continue wrapping the lock of hair to form a large circle on the spongy base. Insert pins along the circle to secure in place.

10. Draw a second lock of hair below the first lock and mist with holding spray.

11. Using tail combs for support, draw the hair downwards then forwards to form a large circle. Draw the hair around to form a circle that overlaps the first circle.

12. Continue wrapping the lock of hair around, using tail combs for support, then replacing the tail combs with pins.

13. Draw a third lock of hair below the second lock and mist with holding spray. Draw the hair downwards and forwards to form another circle that overlaps the second circle.

14. Continue wrapping the lock of hair around, using tail combs for support, then replacing the tail combs with pins.

15. Brush the loose hair with a round brush to make outward curls and blow dry.

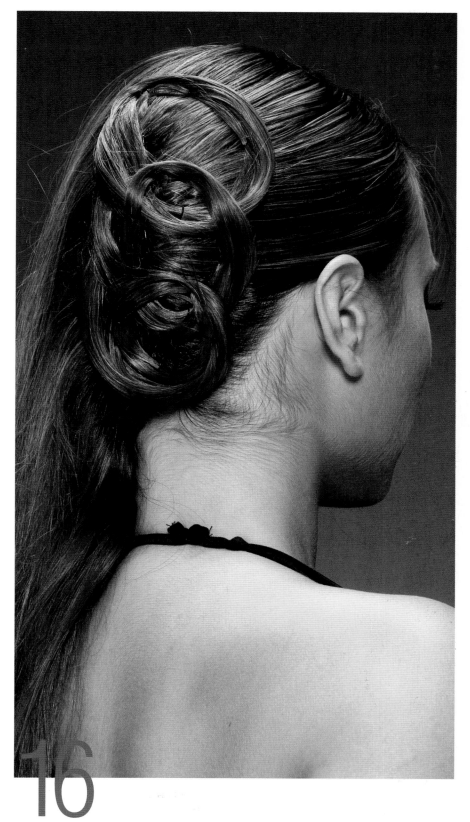

16

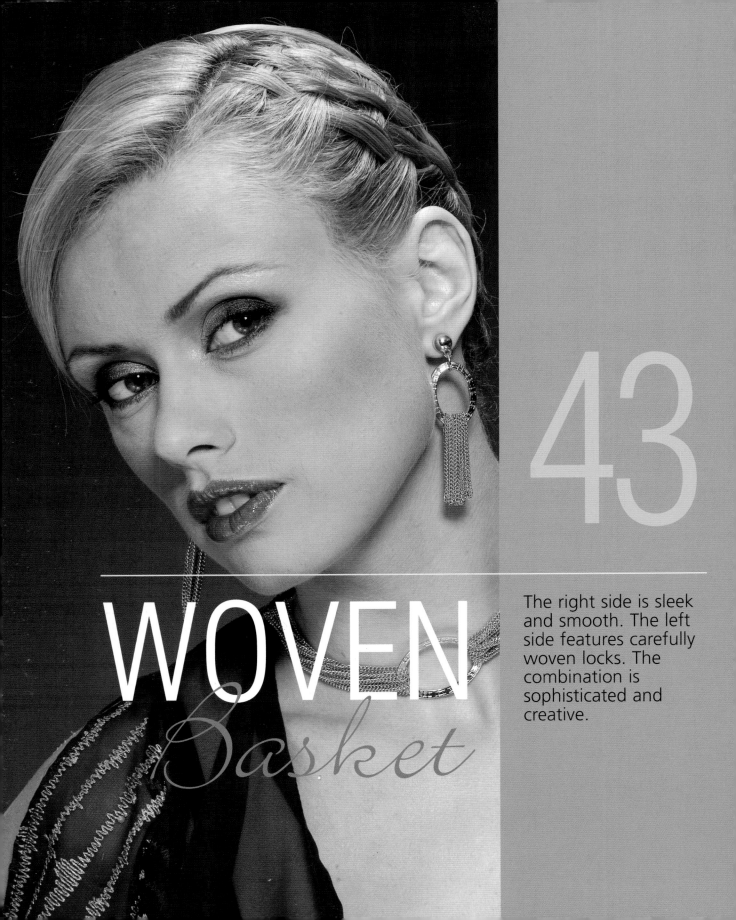

WOVEN *Basket*

43

The right side is sleek and smooth. The left side features carefully woven locks. The combination is sophisticated and creative.

1. Wash and blow dry hair straight. Make a middle part from the brow to the nape of the neck. Hold the hair to the left of the part with a clip. Backcomb the hair on the right side of the part, from the crown to the nape of the neck.

2. Weave a tail comb in and out of the hair on the left side of the part, starting at the forehead and moving towards the crown, to draw four locks of hair upwards.

3. Hold up the locks of hair closest to the brow with one hand and the other locks with the other hand.

4. Draw the lock of hair at the brow backwards while holding the three locks upwards. Secure to the spongy base with a hairpin.

5. Brush the other locks of hair downwards, and over the lock that is pinned at the back of the head.

6. Weave a tail comb in and out of the hair again to lift opposite locks of hair.

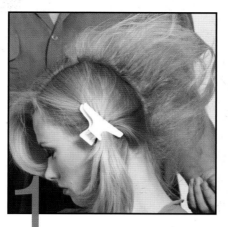

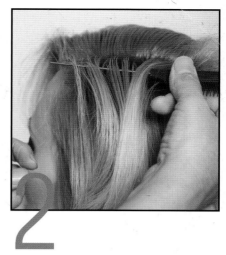

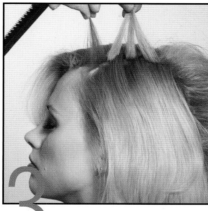

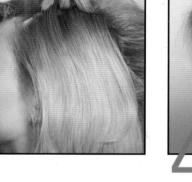

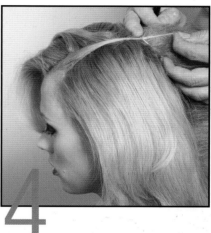

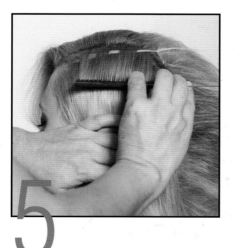

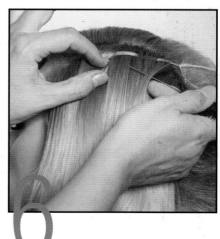

7. Lift the four locks of hair above the tail comb upwards, and brush the other locks of hair downwards.

8. Draw the lock of hair at the brow backwards and secure to the spongy base with a hairpin. Comb the other locks of hair downwards over the lock that is pinned at the back

9. Weave a tail comb in and out of the hair again to draw up opposite locks of hair.

10. Continue in this manner to make a woven surface on the left side of the head. Secure the weave with a seam of pins at the edge of the spongy base.

11. Move to the hair on the right side of the part. Hold the bangs with a clip and brush the rest of the hair backwards.

12. Twist the hair over a finger to form an upright twist that conceals the seam of pins.

13. Secure the twist with hair-pins, leaving the ends of hair loose and extending from the top of the twist.

14. Brush the ends of the hair upwards so that they are smooth at the top of the head.

15. Brush the bangs backwards and tuck behind the right ear.

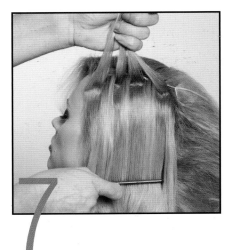

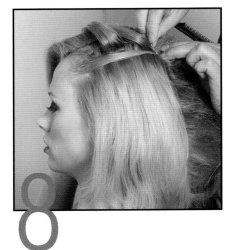

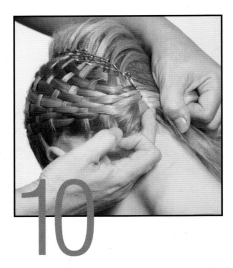

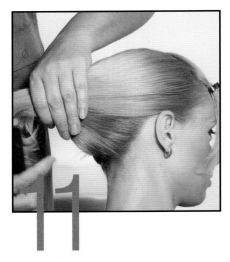

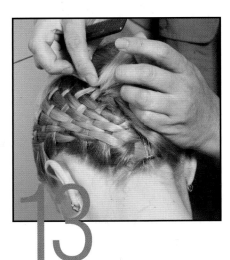

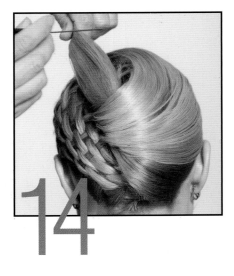

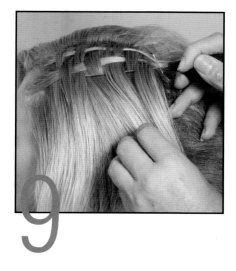

9

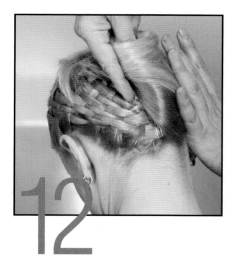

12

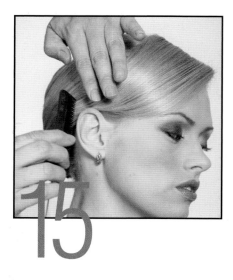

15

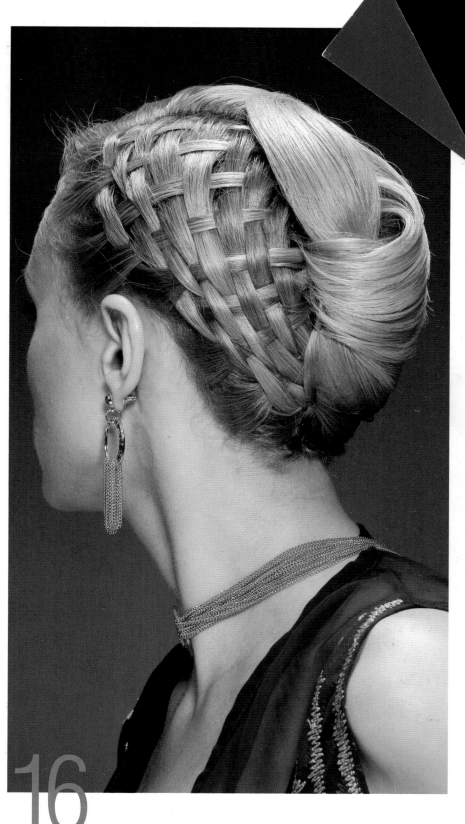

16

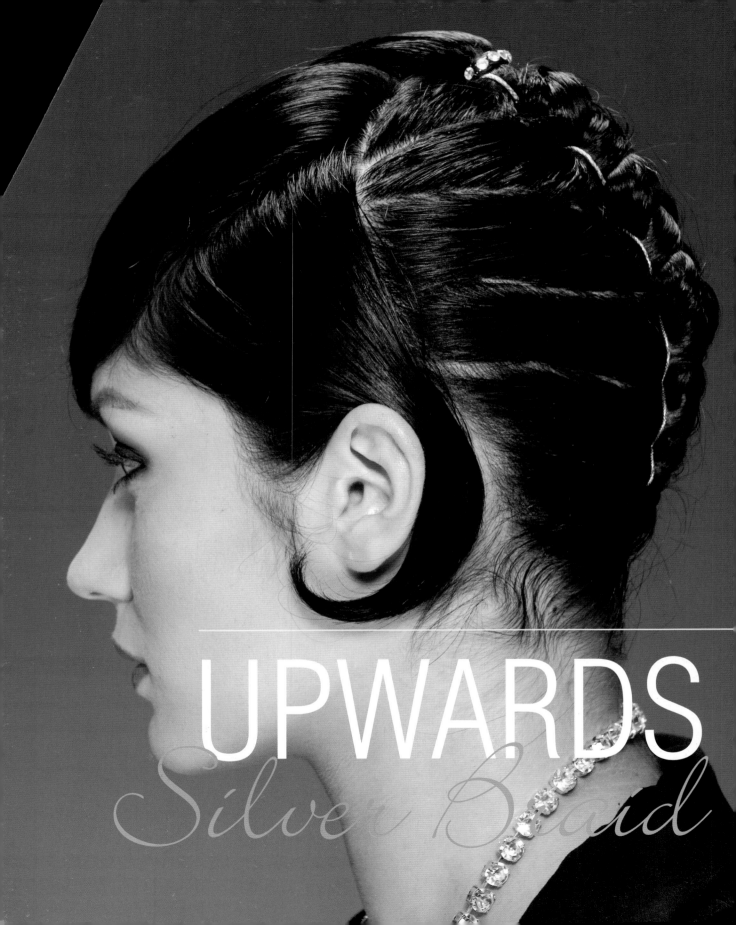

UPWARDS

Silver Braid

44

This backwards braid is tidy, distinct, and sure to set people wondering just how it was made. Use a shiny ribbon to maximize the effect.

1. Wash and blow dry hair straight. Bend over so that the bottom hair can be reached comfortably. Mist with holding spray, and brush the hair upwards. Make a horizontal part about 1 inch above the nape of the neck. Plait the hair in this section into a braid and secure with a bobby pin.

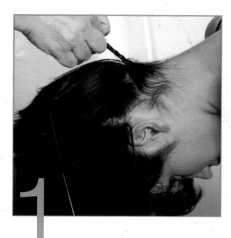

2. Lay a silver ribbon over the braid and secure with a bobby pin. Make a horizontal part 1 inch above the previous part. Divide the hair below the part into two sections, so that the braid lies in the middle.

3. Plait a braid using these two sections and the braid.

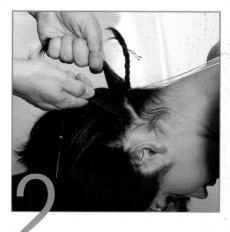

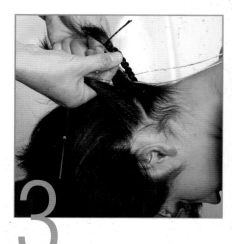

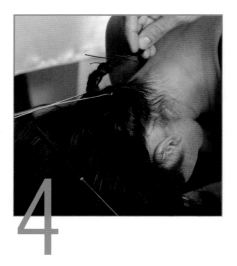

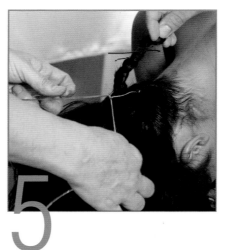

4. Remove the pin from the first braid and use it to secure this braid.

5. Draw the ends of the ribbon to the top of the braid and tie in a knot.

6. Make a horizontal part about 1 inch above the previous part, from the top of the right ear to the top of the left ear. Divide the hair below the part into two sections, so that the braid lies in the middle.

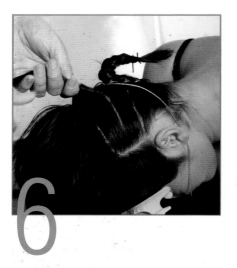

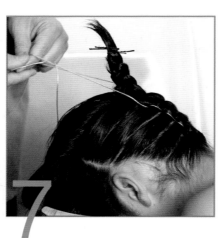

7. Remove the pin from the first braid, when necessary, and use it to secure this braid. Draw the ribbon to the top of the braid, and tie in a knot.

8. Make another part above the previous part. Divide the hair into two sections and plait another braid, integrating the previous braid in the middle. Secure the new braid with the pin, and tie the ribbon in a knot on top of the braid.

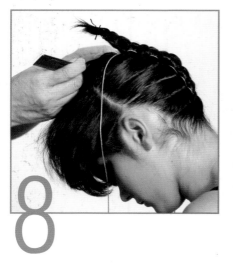

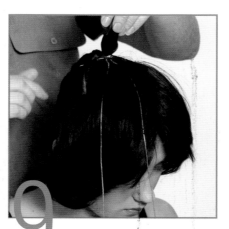

9. Continue braiding the hair upwards in this manner until the braid reaches the crown. Secure with an elastic band close to the roots. Tie the ribbon in a knot and trim the ends.

10. Brush the ends of the braid forwards, integrating them into the front hair.

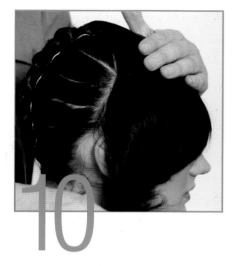

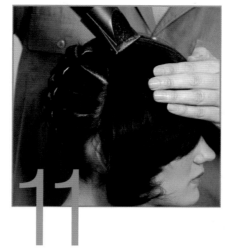

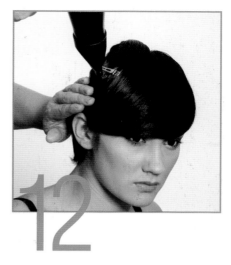

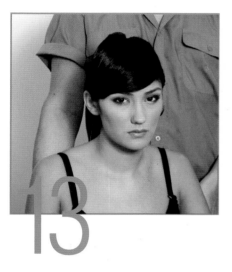

11. Mist with holding spray and blow dry the hair forwards.

12. Brush the front hair backwards and to the right so that the hair flows behind the right ear.

13. Brush the hair so that it is sleek and smooth.

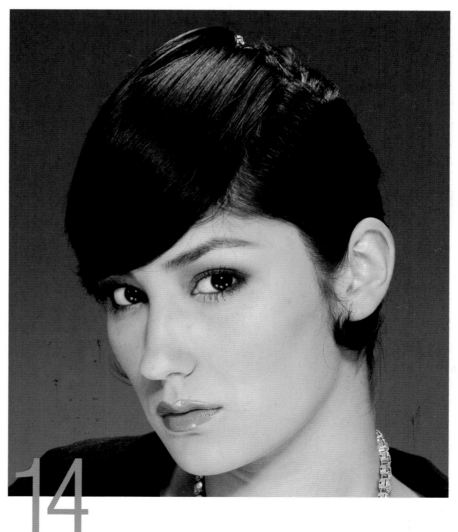

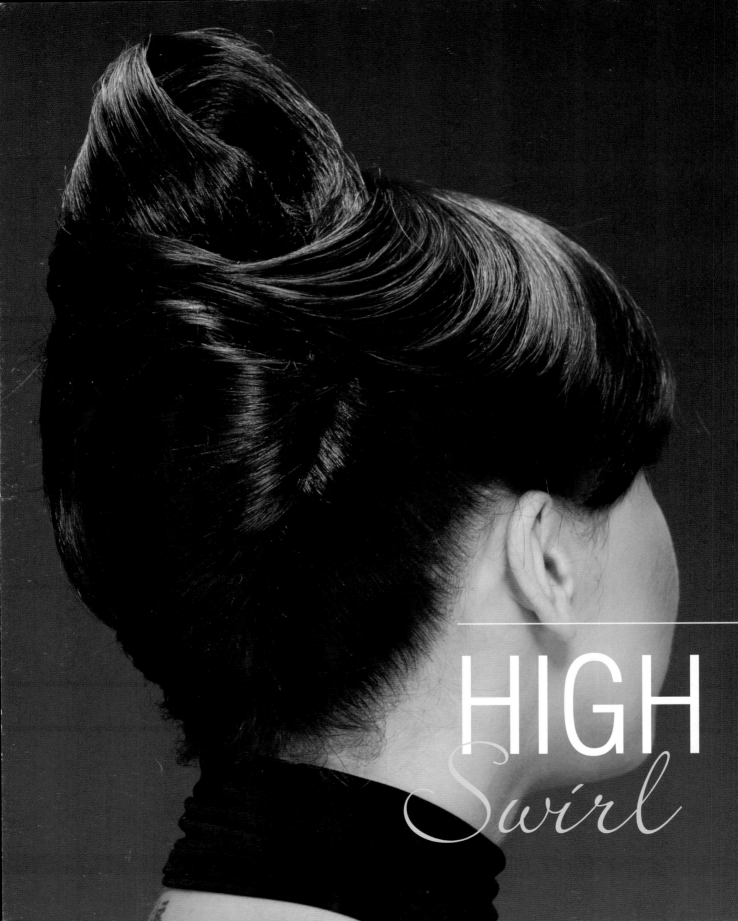

HIGH

Swirl

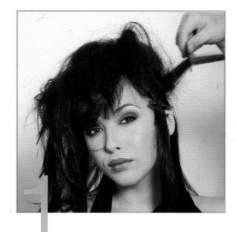

1. Wash and blow dry hair straight. Divide the hair into front and back sections with a part that extends from ear to ear over the crown. Backcomb the hair in the back section to make a spongy base. Make a left side part in the front hair, and hold the hair on either side of the part with clips.

2. Brush the back hair on the right side upwards. Secure with a seam of pins near the middle of the head.

3. Brush the back hair on the left side upwards and back-wards, drawing it over the seam of pins.

4. Twist the hair over a finger to form an upright twist that conceals the seam of pins.

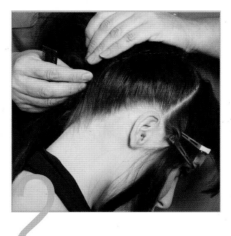

45

Draw hair upwards and around to add elevation in this style. An excellent design for topping off a simple outfit.

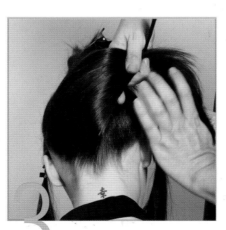

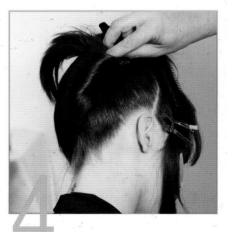

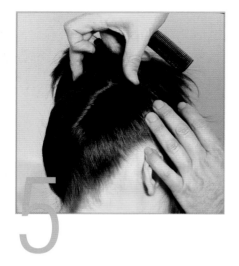

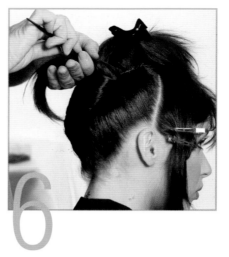

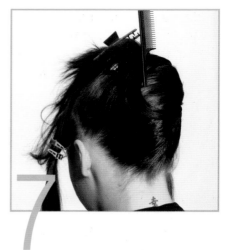

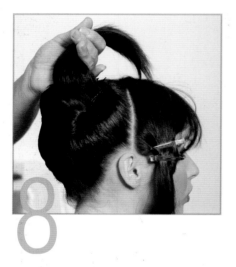

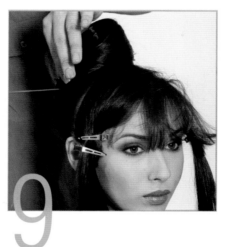

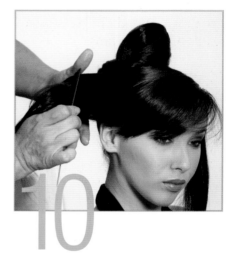

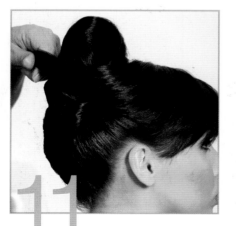

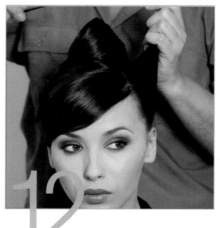

5. Secure with hairpins, leaving the ends loose, and extending from the top of the twist.

6. Divide the loose ends into top and bottom sections. Hold the top section with a clip and brush the bottom section into a flat strip.

7. Curve the strip in a C-shaped arc over the twist. Use tail combs for support, then mist with holding spray.

8. Brush the top section of hair extending from the twist forwards and brush into a wide strip.

9. Draw the ends of the strip towards the back to form a cone on the top of the head. Secure the cone with hairpins.

10. Release the right front hair from the clip and brush it downwards and backwards.

11. Mist the hair with holding spray and sweep it upwards at the back of the head, drawing it around the cone.

12. Release the left front hair and brush it upwards and backwards.

13. Tuck the hair behind the cone, above the arc of hair.

14. Secure with a tail comb, then secure with hairpins. Mist with holding spray.

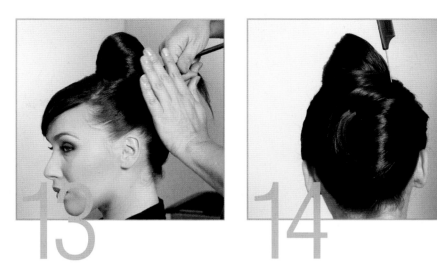

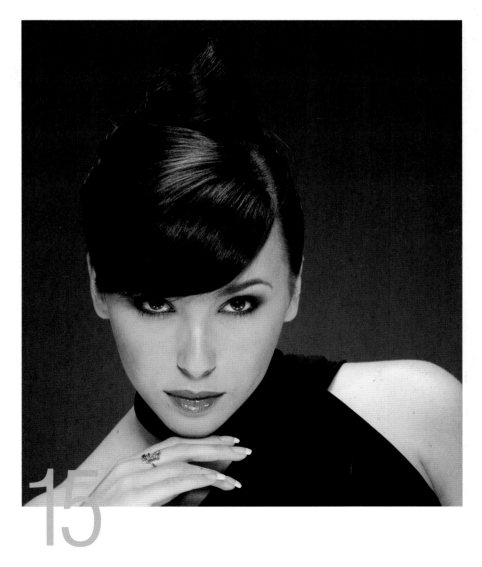

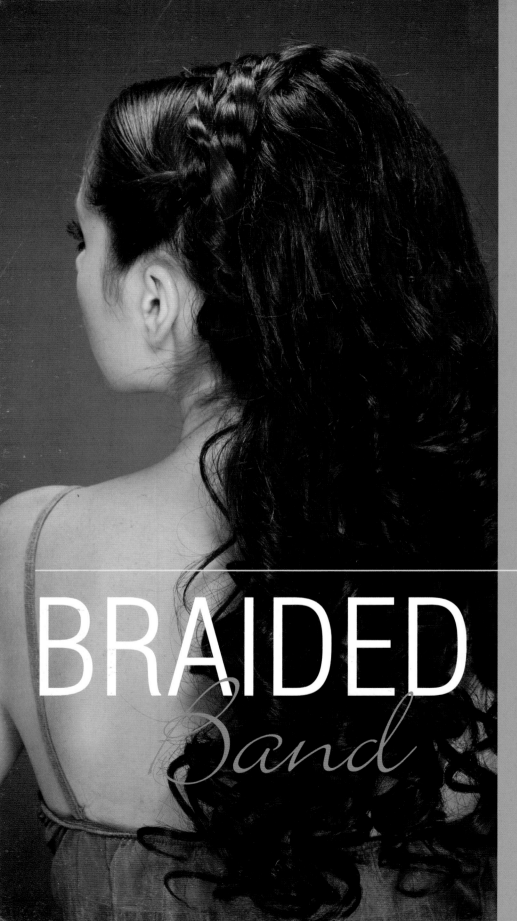

BRAIDED
Band

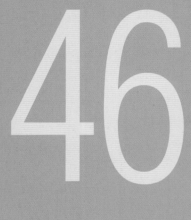

46

Simple and flowing, this style uses natural hair to form a twisted hair band. A curled hair extension is added to increase length and romance.

1. Wash and blow dry hair curly. Divide the hair into front and back sections with a part that extends from ear to ear over the crown. Backcomb the hair behind the part at the crown. Make a middle part in the front hair.

2. Backcomb a rectangular section at the top of the head to make a spongy base.

3. Select a long hair extension and curl the ends into ringlets with a curling iron. Separate each curl into three or four locks.

4. Sew the extension onto the spongy base using a blunt needle and thick thread.

5. Lift the extension and divide the natural hair underneath into left and right sections.

6. Divide the hair on the right into two sections. Twist the sections together to form a rope.

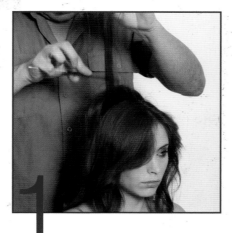

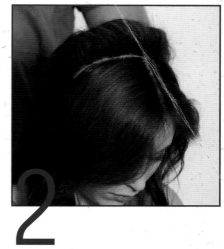

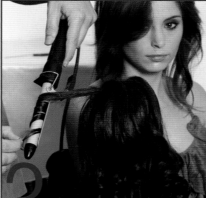

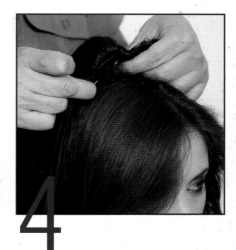

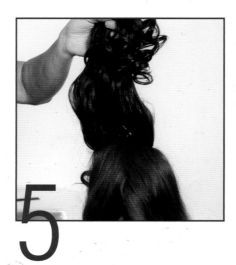

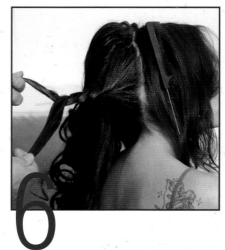

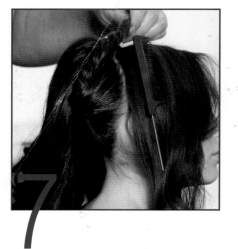

7

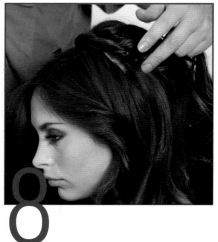

8

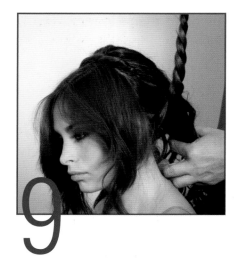

9

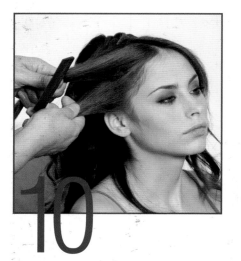

10

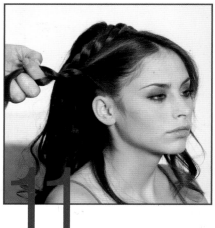

11

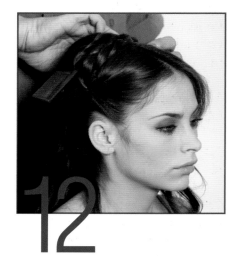

12

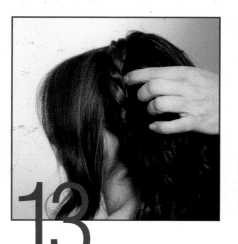

13

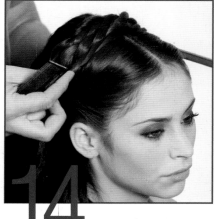

14

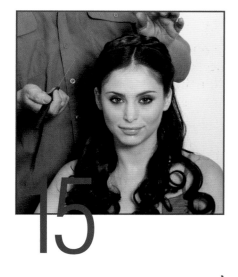

15

7. Roll the rope inwards and draw the end to the crown.

8. Draw the end over the top of the head, concealing the stitches that hold the extension. Secure with a hairpin on the left side of the extension.

9. Divide the hair on the left into two sections and twist together to form a rope.

10. Twist the rope inwards and draw the end upwards, over the top of the head and beside the first rope. Secure with a hairpin on the right side of the extension.

11. Divide the front right hair into top and bottom sections.

12. Twist the sections upwards to form a rope.

13. Draw the rope upwards and over the head. Support with a tail comb, then secure on the left side of the head with hairpins.

14. Repeat on the left side, dividing the hair into two sections and twisting sections together to form a rope. Draw the rope over the head and pin it on the right side.

15. Brush the extension forwards, so that there are curls on both shoulders.

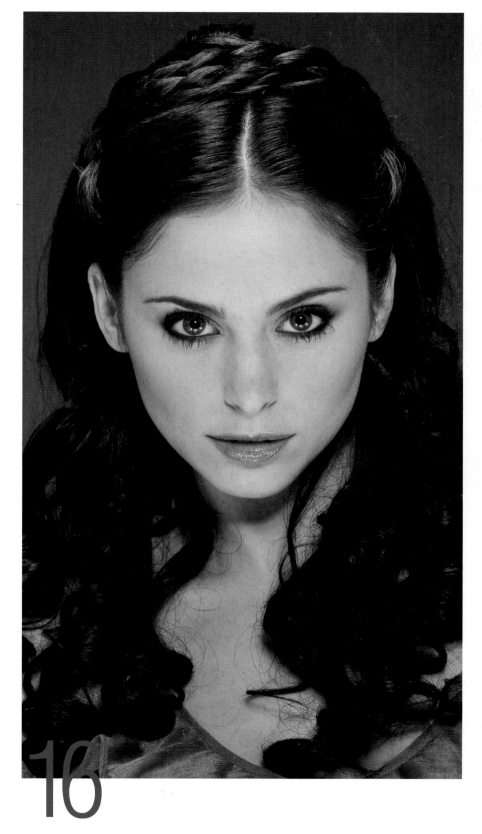

16

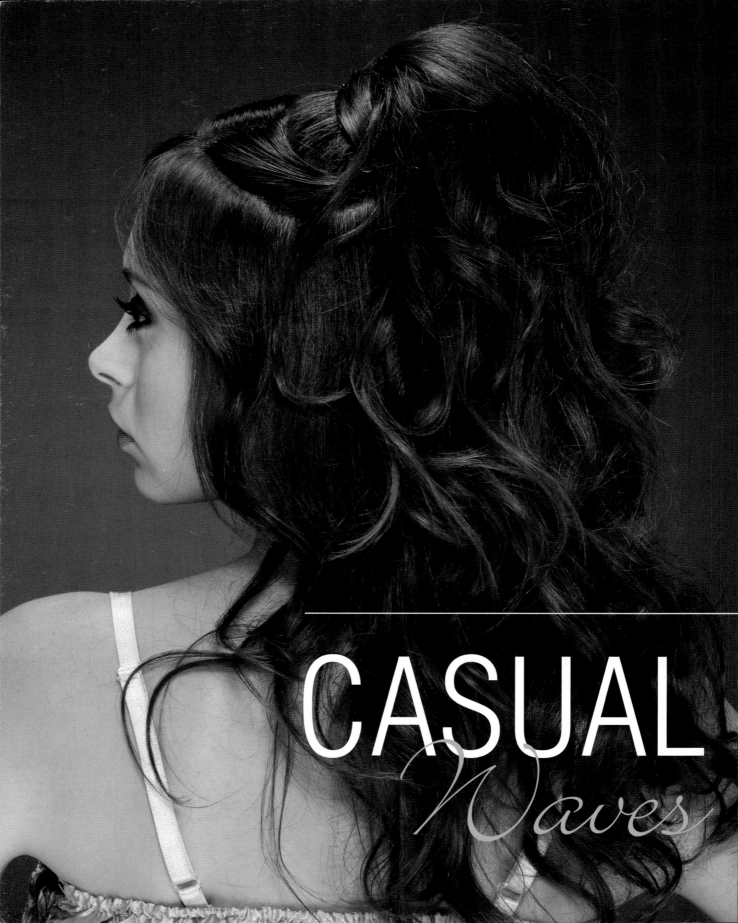

CASUAL *Waves*

47

Sexy and sweet, this hairstyle flows naturally. It uses a few simple techniques that add body and style.

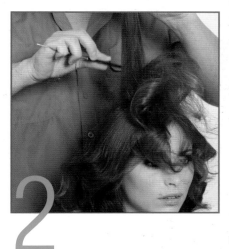

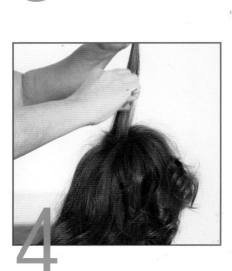

1. Wash and blow dry hair. Curl the hair into loose ringlets with a curling iron.

2. Backcomb the hair at the top of the head.

3. Divide the hair into front and back sections with a part that extends from ear to ear over the crown. Brush back the hair behind the crown and secure with a seam of pins. Divide the front hair with a left side part.

4. Backcomb the hair behind the pins.

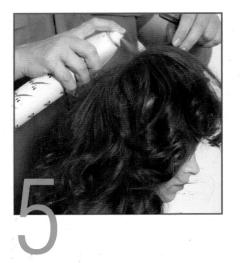 5

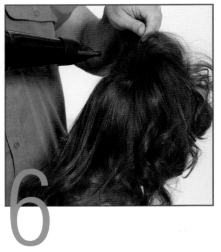 6

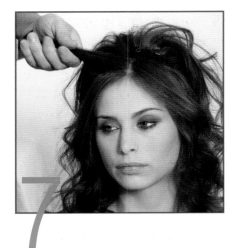 7

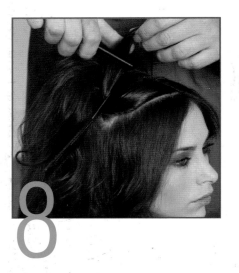 8

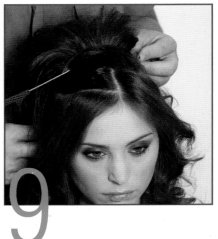 9

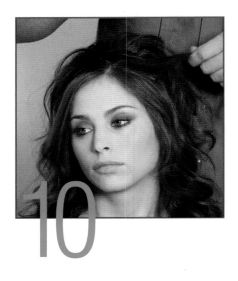 10

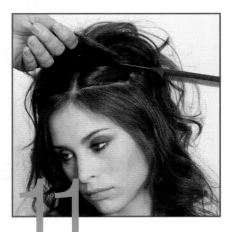 11

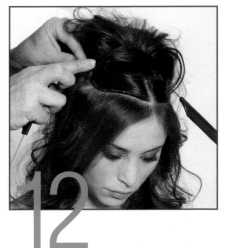 12

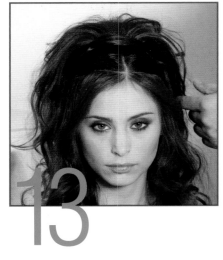 13

5. Mist holding spray at the roots of the backcombed hair.

6. Blow dry the hair at the top of the head on medium heat.

7. Make a triangular part in the right front hair, just in front of the seam of pins.

8. Mist the hair with holding spray and brush it downwards and backwards. Use a tail comb for support, then draw the hair upwards and backwards, towards the left side of the head.

9. Draw the hair over the seam of pins to conceal it and secure on the left side of the pins with a hairpin.

10. Take a similar section of hair on the other side of the part. Mist with holding spray and comb the hair downwards and backwards.

11. Use a tail comb for support, then draw the hair over to the right side of the head, just in front of the previous section.

12. Secure the hair with a pin.

13. Style the hair with your fingers to give it a casual, care-free appearance.

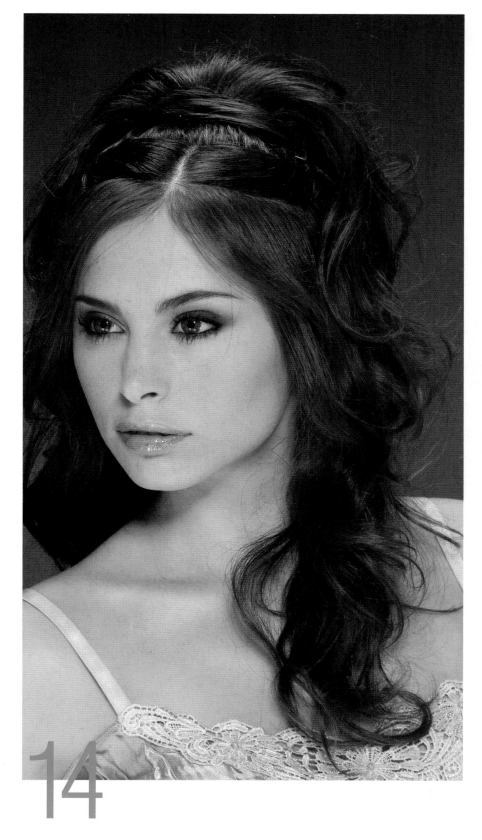

14

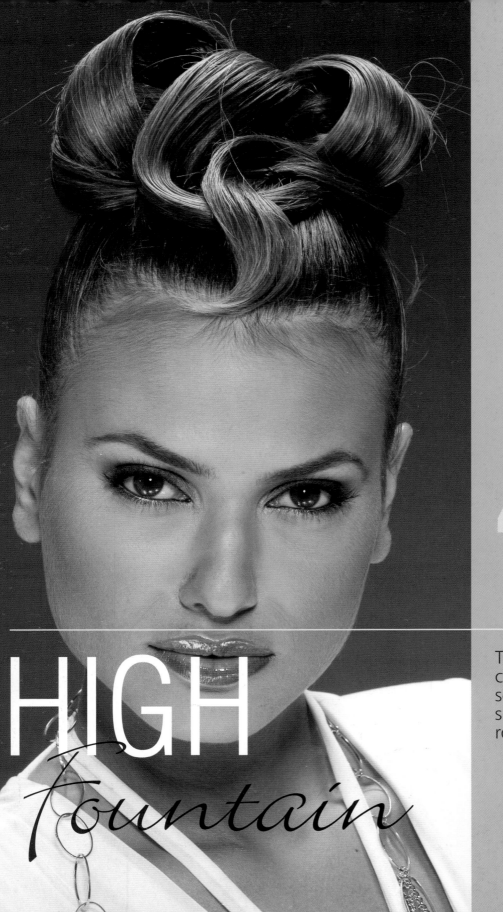

48

This enigmatic design conveys a sense of sophistication, with a subtle touch of romance.

HIGH
Fountain

1. Wash and blow dry hair straight. Gather the hair in a high ponytail at the crown. Draw a lock of hair, brush into a flat strip, and wrap around the base of the ponytail to conceal the elastic band. Divide the ponytail into four sections. Mist the rightmost section with holding spray and blow dry into a flat strip.

2. Roll the strip outwards into a loop. Secure the loop near the base of the ponytail, leaving the ends loose and extending out the back of the loop.

3. Draw the loose ends around the front of the loop on the right side, and through the loop to the back of the head. Use a tail comb for support.

4. Replace the tail comb with hairpins to secure.

5. Mist the front section of the ponytail with holding spray and brush into a flat strip. Draw the strip forwards, then wrap around a tail comb and draw backwards, towards the base of the ponytail.

6. Secure with a hairpin, leaving the ends loose and forwards.

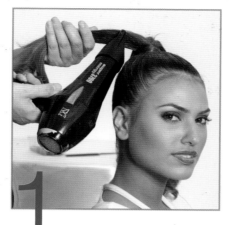
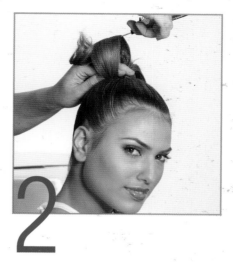
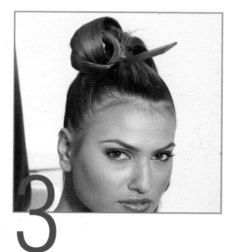
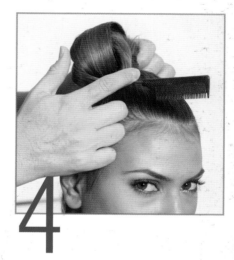
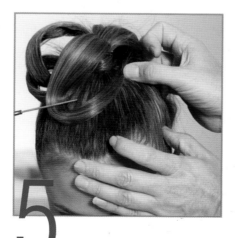
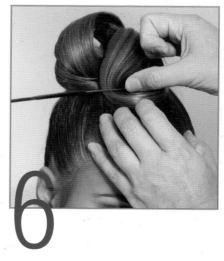

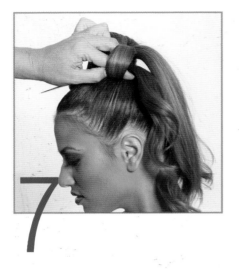

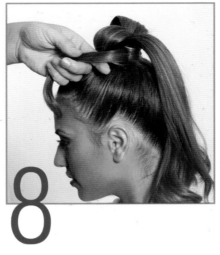

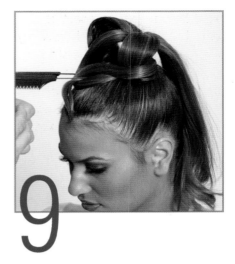

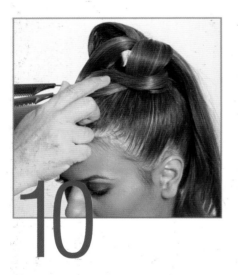

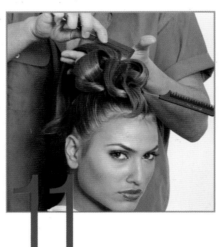

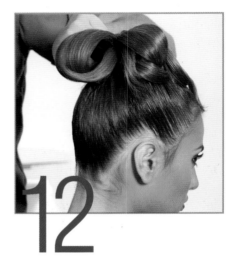

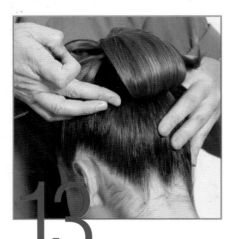

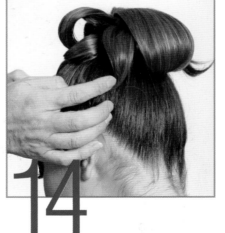

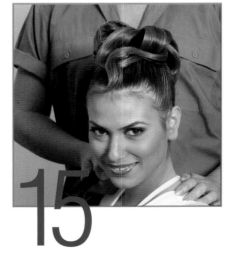

7. Mist the leftmost section with holding spray and blow dry into a flat strip. Roll the strip outwards to form a large loop and secure near the base of the ponytail, leaving the ends loose and extending out the back of the loop.

8. Draw the loose ends around the front of the loop on the left side.

9. Use tail combs to support the hair and gently curve it over the front of the head, so that the ends lie gently on the forehead.

10. Secure the hair with a hairpin.

11. Mist the back section of the ponytail with holding spray and brush into a flat strip.

12. Roll the hair downwards to form a loop, leaving the ends loose.

13. Draw the ends out from either side of the loop.

14. Massage styling mousse onto the ends of the hair and shape into small leaves on either side of the head.

15. Mist with holding spray to hold the loops in place.

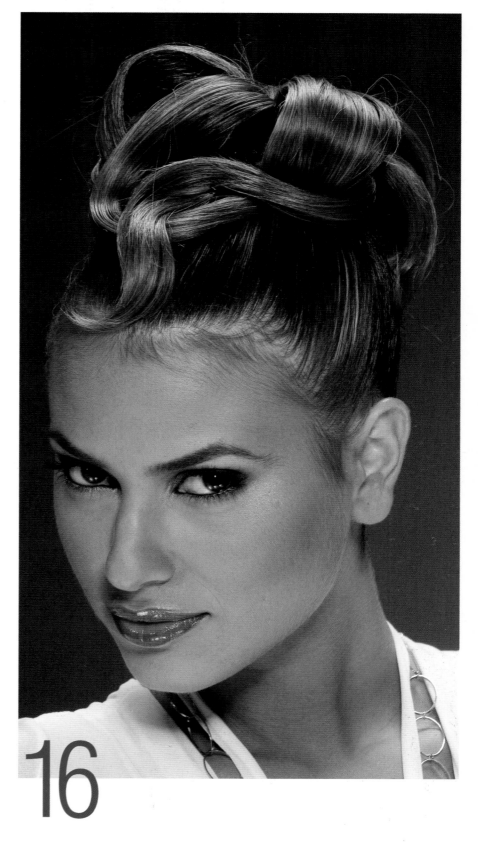

16

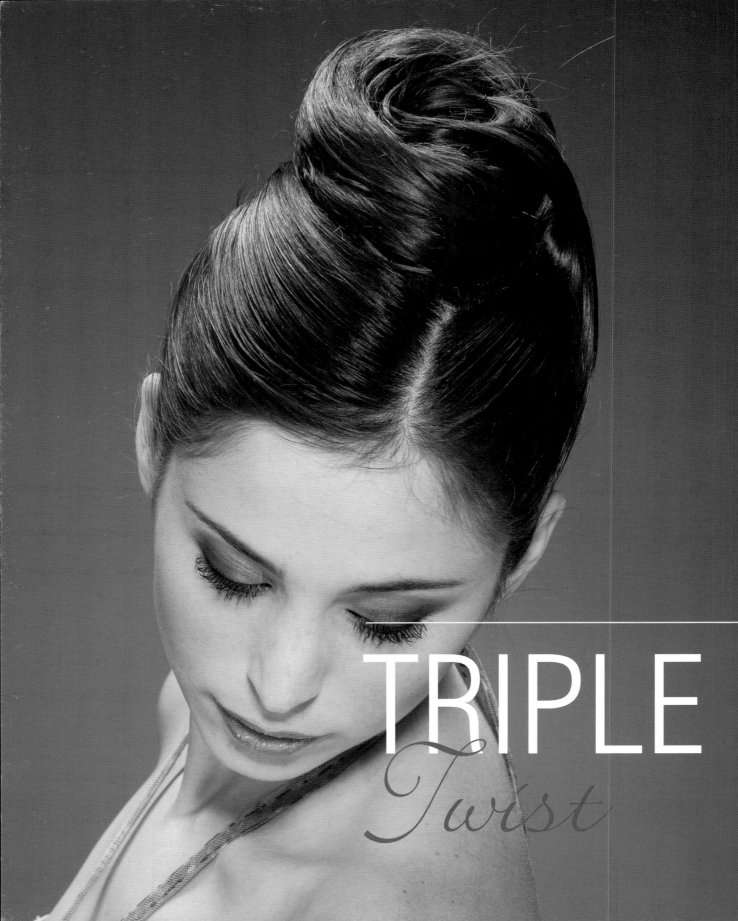

TRIPLE

Twist

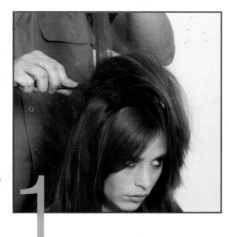

49

The central twist in this design increases height. Two side twists add a delicate touch of elegance.

1. Wash and blow dry hair straight. Divide the hair into front and back sections by making a part from ear to ear over the crown. Divide the front hair with a left side part. Backcomb the top of the back hair.

2. Continue backcombing the hair until you have a spongy base that extends from ear to ear.

3. Brush back the top of the backcombed hair and secure with a seam of pins behind the crown.

4. Brush the hair at the right side, from the crown to the bottom of the ear, upwards. Secure with a seam of pins that is perpendicular to the first seam of pins. Mist with holding spray and blow dry.

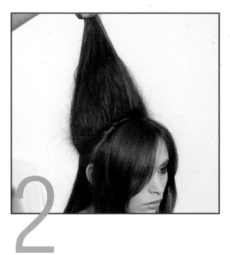

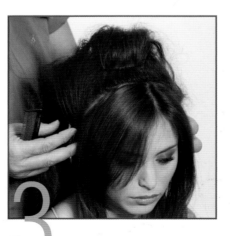

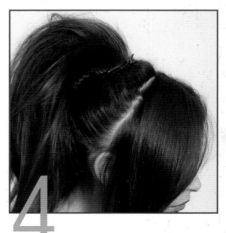

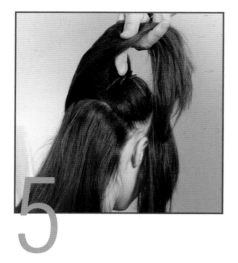

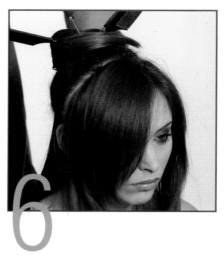

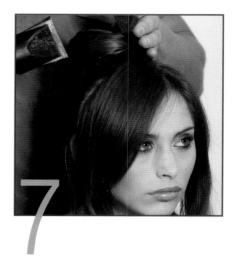

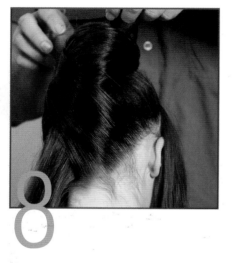

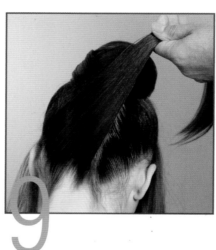

5. Brush a similar section of hair on the left side upwards and twist over the seam of pins.

6. Using tail combs for support, wrap the hair over the seam of pins, twisting it forwards to make a cone.

7. Insert hairpins to secure the cone, then mist with holding spray and blow dry.

8. Divide the hair at the back of the head into right and left sections. Brush the right section upwards and towards the left, wrapping it upwards around the base of the cone. Draw the ends to the front of the head, and tuck them into the cone.

9. Brush the left section upwards and towards the right.

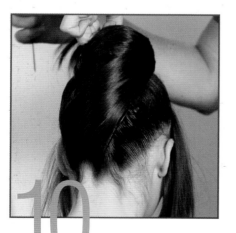

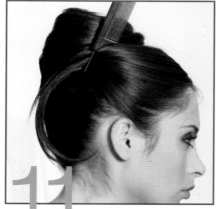

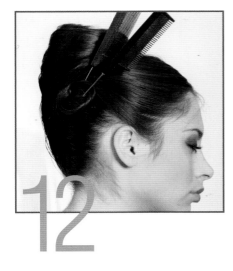

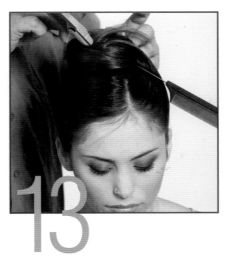

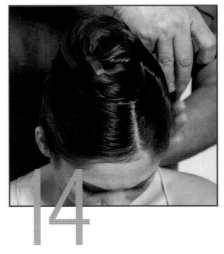

10. Wrap the hair around the base of the cone, drawing the ends to the front and tucking them around the cone to form an envelope of hair at the back of the head.

11. Brush the right front hair backwards. Draw it upwards along the cone, using a tail comb for support.

12. Coil the hair into a flat Figure 6. Support with tail combs, then secure with hairpins.

13. Brush the front left hair backwards. Use a tail comb for support and draw the hair over the cone, tucking the ends into the top of the cone.

14. Coil the hair inside the cone, using tail combs for support. Secure with hairpins and mist with holding spray.

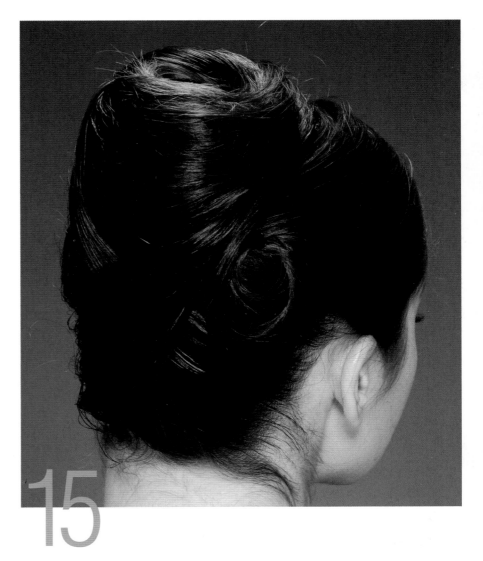

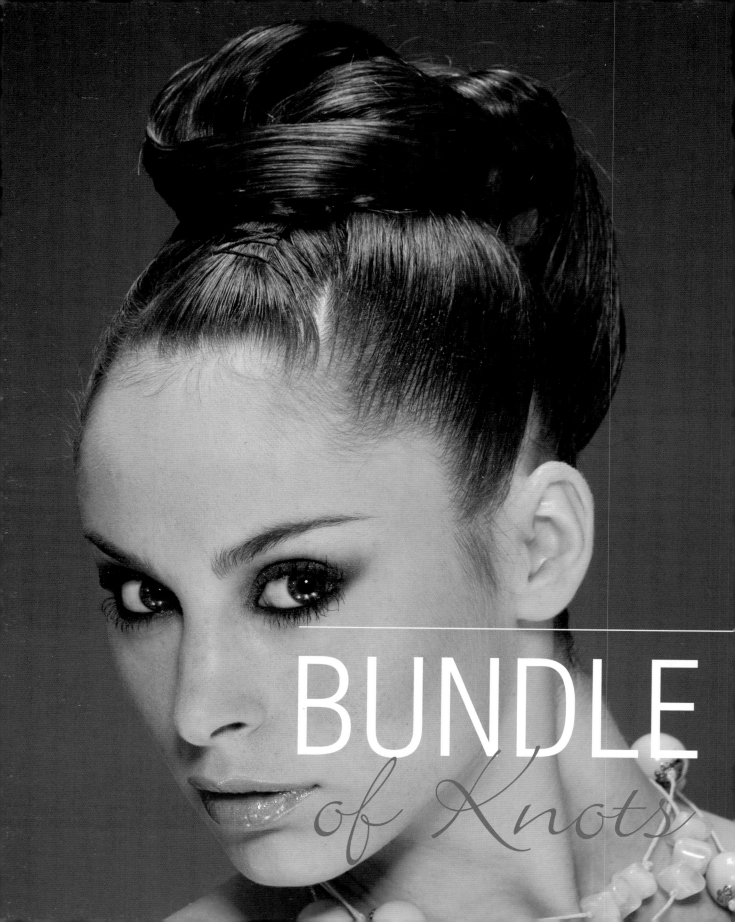

BUNDLE
of Knots

1. Wash and blow dry hair straight. Gather all of the hair in a high ponytail at the top of the head. Draw a lock of hair from the ponytail, mist with holding spray, and brush into a flat strip. Wrap the strip around the base of the ponytail to conceal the elastic band. Select a long hair extension.

2. Sew the extension just above the ponytail with a blunt needle and thick thread.

3. Wrap the thread around a 2-inch section of hair in front of the extension. Continue wrapping the thread around this section of hair, from the ponytail to the brow and back again. Tie the thread in a knot close to the extension.

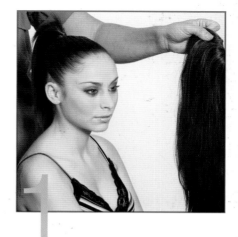

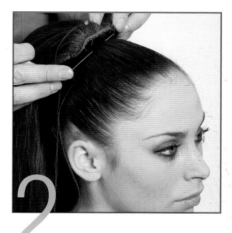

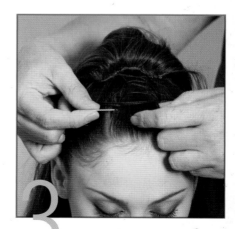

50

Who would have thought knotty hair could be so attractive? The knots are extra thick in this design, thanks to the long hair extension.

4. Divide the extension into right and left sections.

5. Draw the natural ponytail forwards between the two sections of the extension.

6. Mist the natural ponytail with holding spray and brush into a flat strip. Fold the strip forwards, securing it with hairpins to the threaded area at the top. Draw the ends to the left side of the head.

7. Wrap the ends behind the extension and secure with pins.

8. Brush the two sections of the extension into flat strips.

9. Tie the strips in a knot at the back of the head.

10. Tie another knot after the first knot.

11. Draw one strip downwards and to the right. Secure with a bobby pin close to the second knot.

12. Coil the end of the strip into a flat Figure 6 and secure with a pin.

13. Coil the hair on the left side into a flat Figure 6.

14. Secure below the first flat Figure 6 and secure with pins.

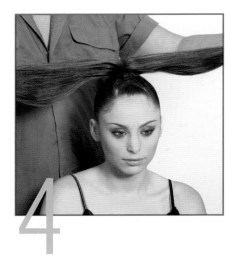
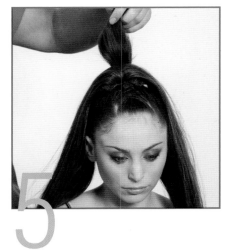
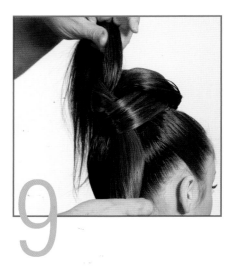
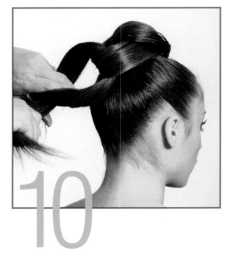
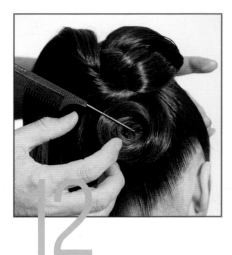
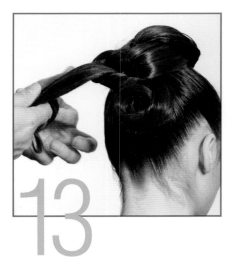

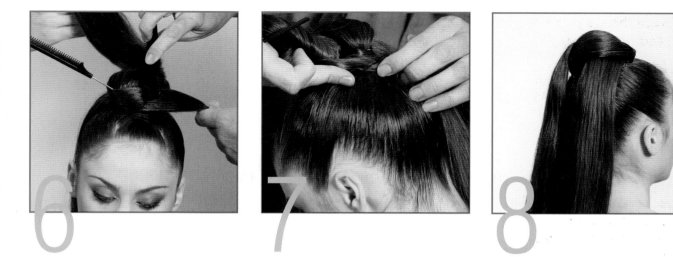

6

7

8

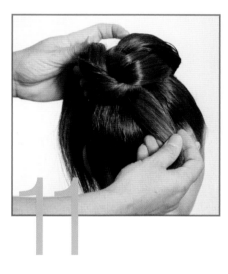

11

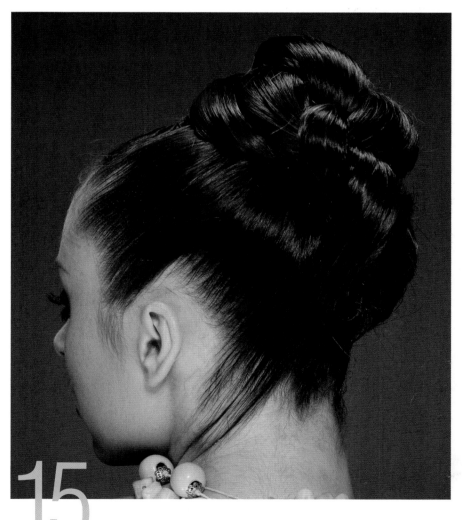

15

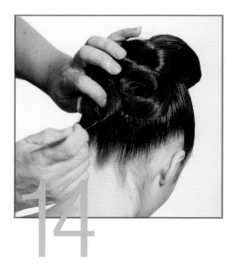

14

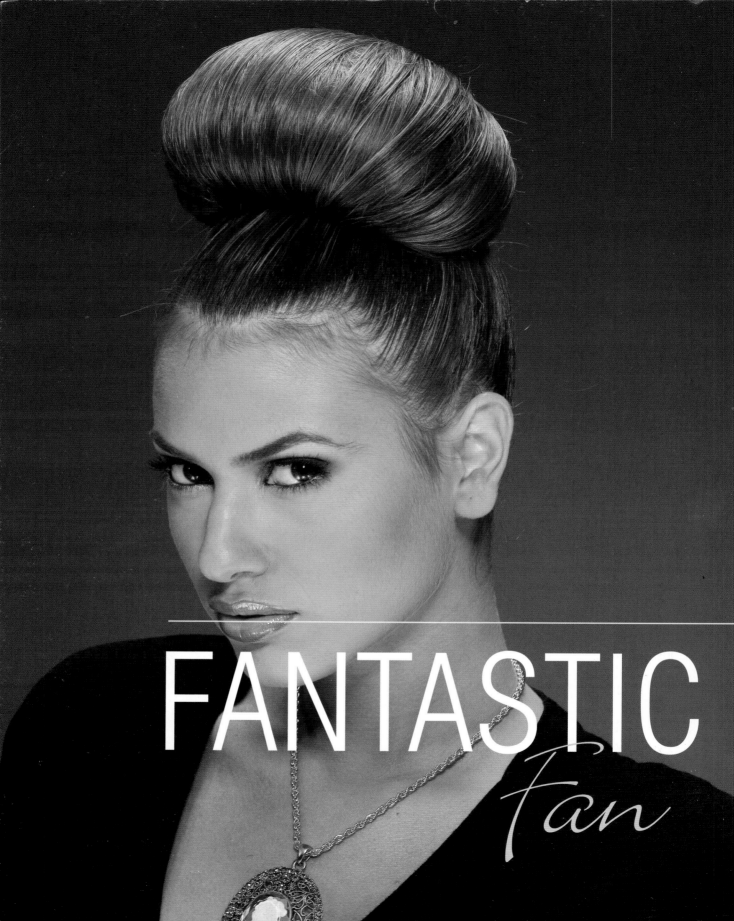

FANTASTIC *Fan*

51

High and exotic, this hairstyle is sure to attract attention in even the most crowded of rooms. Prepare to be noticed.

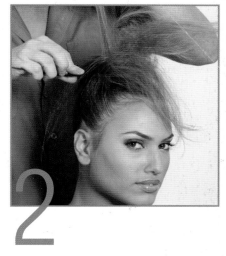

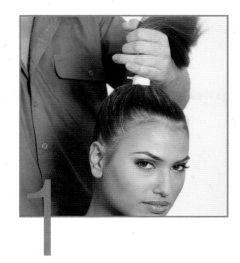

1. Wash and blow dry hair straight. Gather the hair in a high ponytail at the crown.

2. Draw a lock of hair from the ponytail and brush into a flat strip. Wrap the lock around the base of the ponytail to conceal the elastic band. Backcomb the rest of the ponytail.

3. Backcomb the entire ponytail.

4. Brush the ponytail forwards and mist with holding spray.

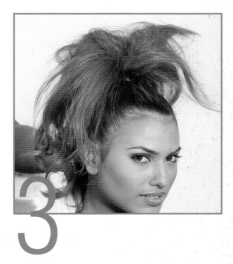

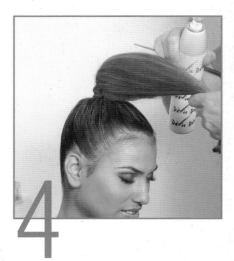

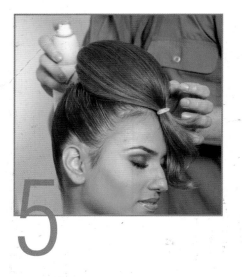

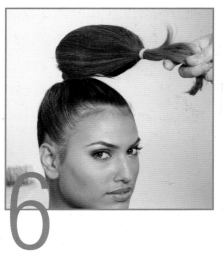

5. Wrap an elastic band near the end of the ponytail to make a closed ponytail. The second elastic band should be in line with the brow.

6. Lift the ponytail upwards and forwards. Roll the ponytail forwards to form a large loop.

7. Secure the loop at the top of the head with hairpins.

8. Draw the ponytail open on either side to make a fan at the top of the head.

9. Insert hairpins on either side of the fan to secure

10. Carefully smooth out the fan with a tail comb.

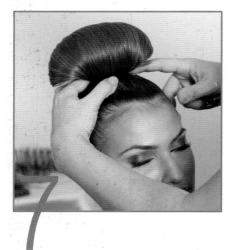

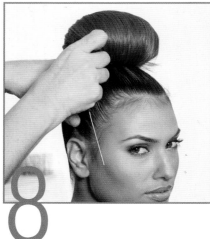

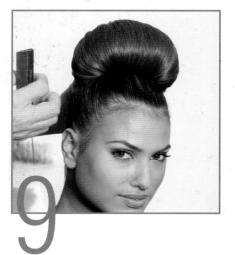

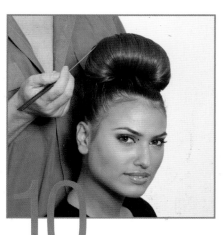

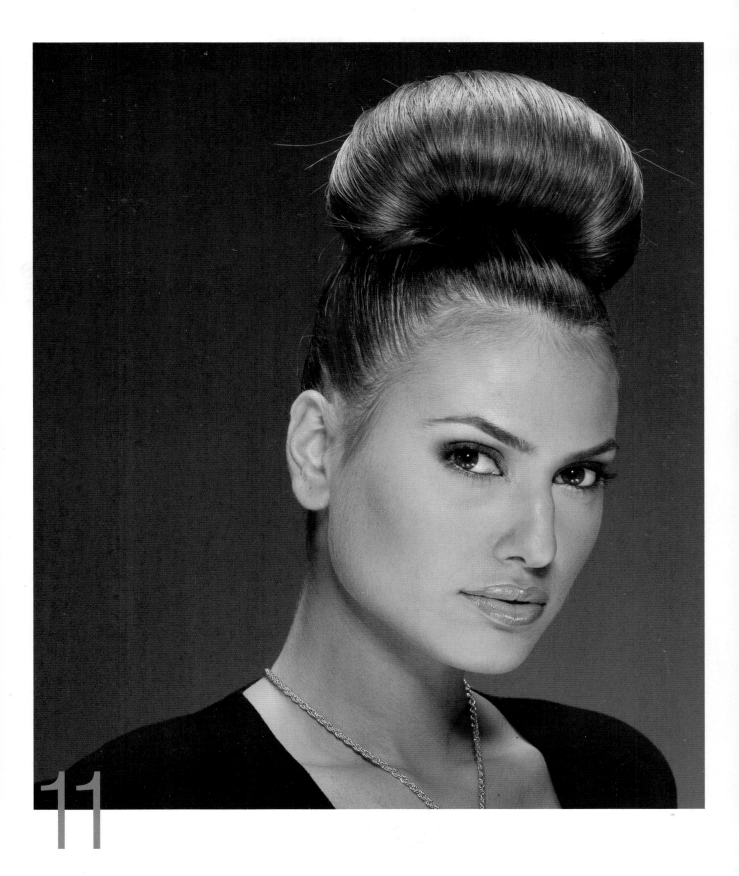

11

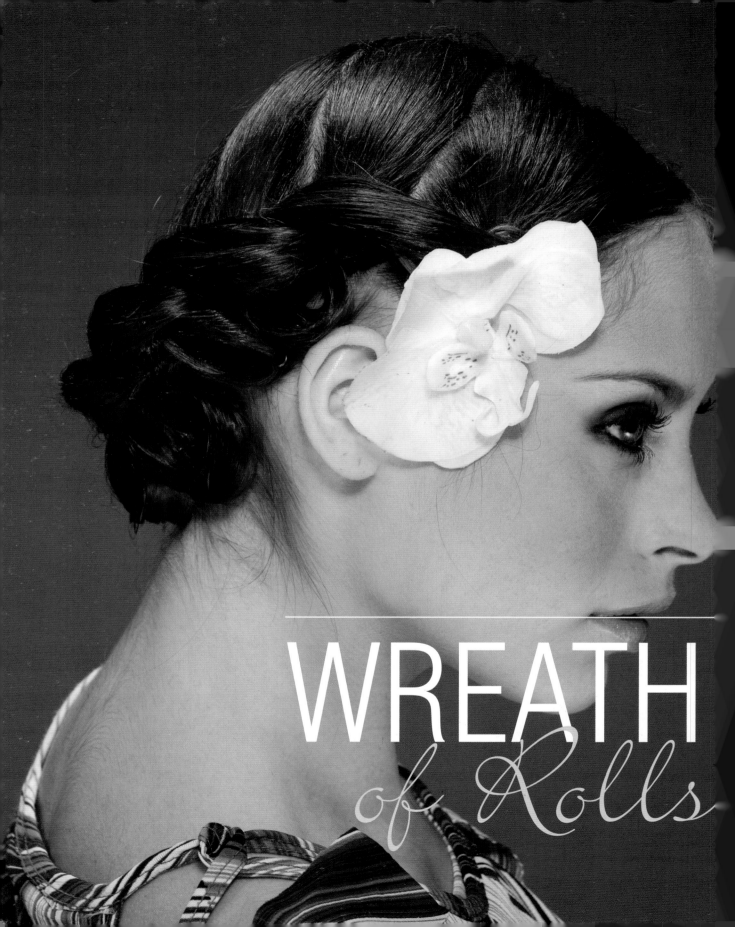

WREATH
of Rolls

52

Wrap yourself in rolls using the simple technique described in this style. Divide each section carefully, since even parts add to the charm.

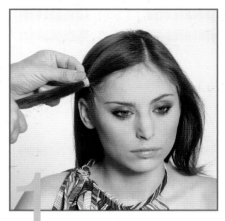

1. Wash and blow dry hair straight. Make a left side part from the brow to the crown. Gather hair from a 2-inch section of hair on the right side of the part in a ponytail close to the roots above the right ear. Draw a lock of hair, brush into a flat strip, and wrap around the base of the ponytail to conceal the elastic band.

2. Mark off a 2-inch section of hair just below the first ponytail and gather in another ponytail. Conceal the elastic band with a lock of hair from the ponytail. Repeat to make a total of eight ponytails all around the head.

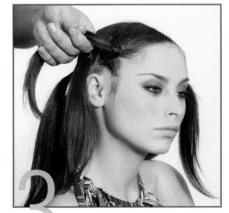

3. Draw the first ponytail on the right backwards.

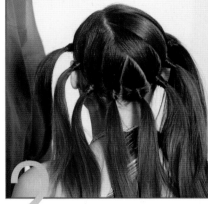

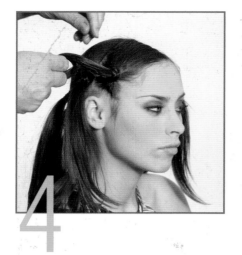

4

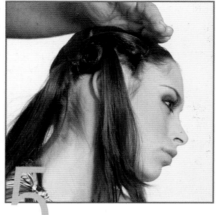

5

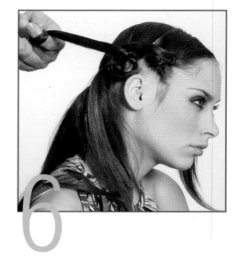

6

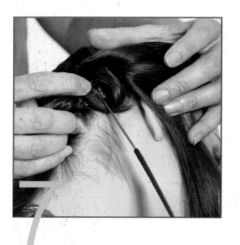

7

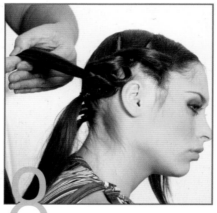

8

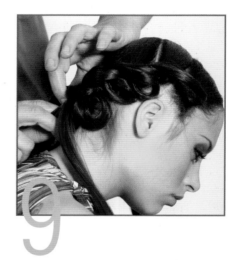

9

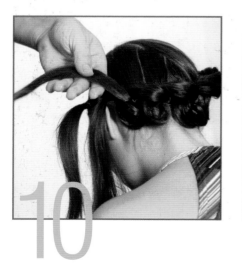

10

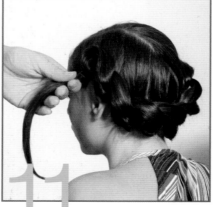

11

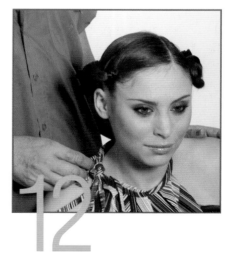

12

4. Coil the ponytail to make a flat Figure 6 behind the second ponytail.

5. Secure with pins behind the second ponytail.

6. Draw the second ponytail backwards and coil to make a flat Figure 6.

7. Draw the Figure 6 behind the third ponytail and secure with pins.

8. Repeat with the third ponytail, coiling it backwards into a flat Figure 6 that lies behind the fourth ponytail.

9. Secure with pins.

10. Continue in this manner working your way around the back of the head and towards the front left side, leaving the first ponytail on the left side loose.

11. Draw the remaining ponytail backwards.

12. Secure with pins beside the flat Figure 6.

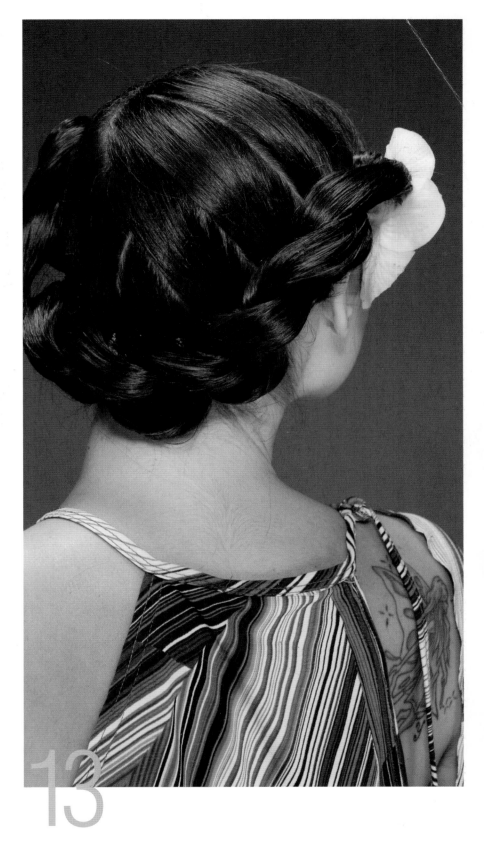

13

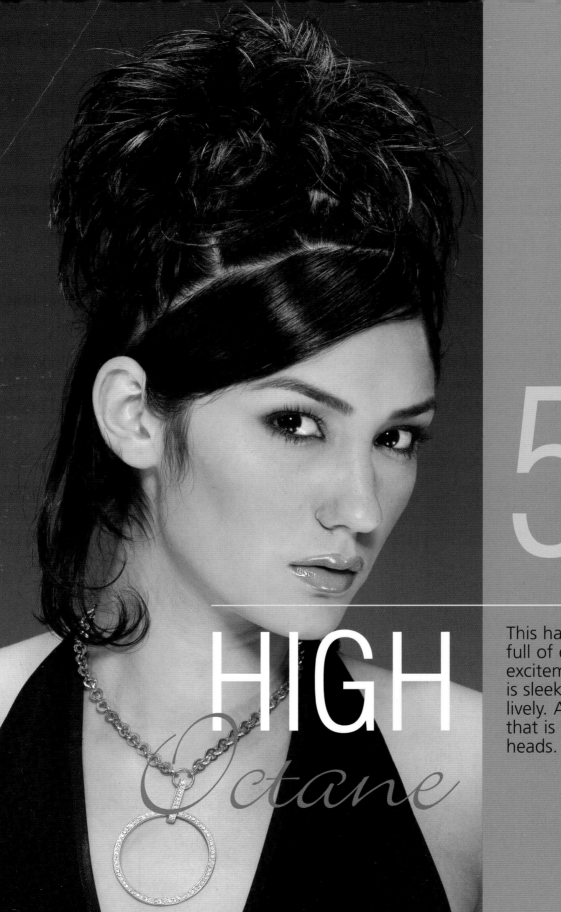

53

HIGH
Octane

This hairstyle is full of energy and excitement. The front is sleek; the back is lively. A dramatic look that is sure to turn heads.

1. Wash and blow dry hair wavy. Backcomb a circular section of hair at the crown.

2. Brush the backcombed hair upwards and secure with a round seam of pins.

3. Take a section of hair in front of the spongy base and twist it backwards.

4. Secure with a bobby pin close to the seam of pins.

5. Take a section of hair to the right of the first section. Twist towards the spongy base and secure with a bobby pin.

6. Take a section of hair to the right of the second section. Draw out a lock and brush towards the face. Twist the rest towards the spongy base and secure with a bobby pin.

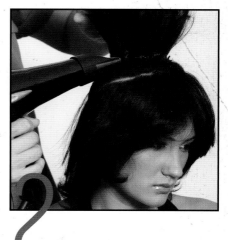

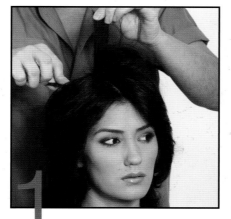

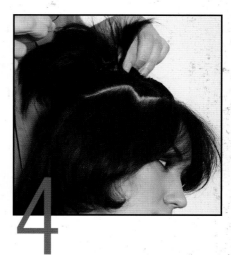

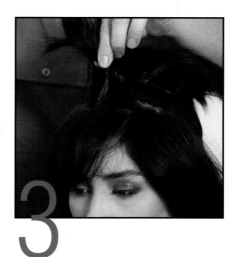

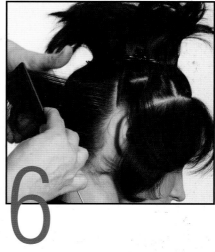

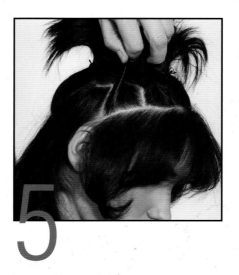

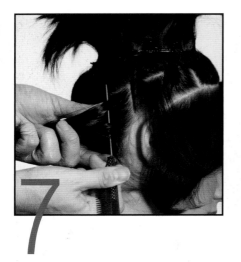

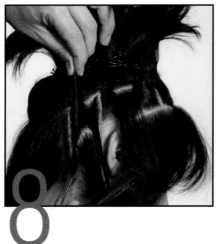

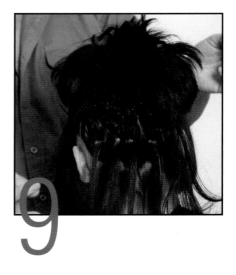

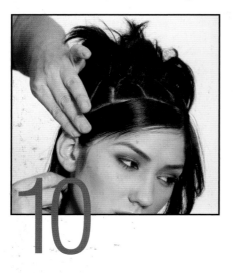

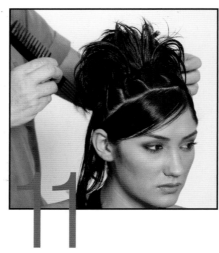

7. Take a fourth section of hair, to the right of the third section. Weave a tail comb in and out to separate two locks of hair. Brush the locks downwards and twist the rest of the hair towards the spongy base.

8. Continue in this manner, working your way around the head, twisting sections of hair towards the spongy base and drawing two locks downwards each time.

9. Repeat until you reach the front left side.

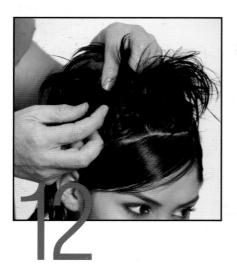

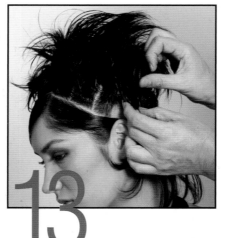

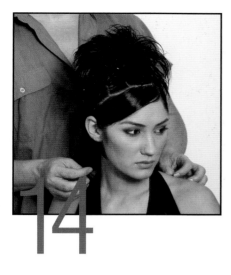

14

10. Make a left side part in the hair. Brush the hair to the right of the part towards the right ear and secure with a bobby pin. Smooth the hair to the left of the part behind the left ear.

11. Use a wide tooth comb to style the hair at the top.

12. Massage liquid spray into the ends of hair at the top.

13. Draw some of the ends downwards to conceal the seam of pins.

14. Orient the rest of the ends to form a fountain at the top of the head.

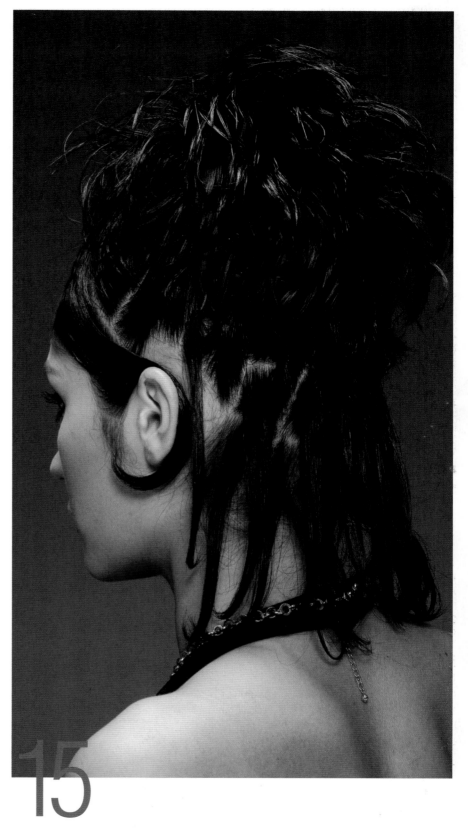

15

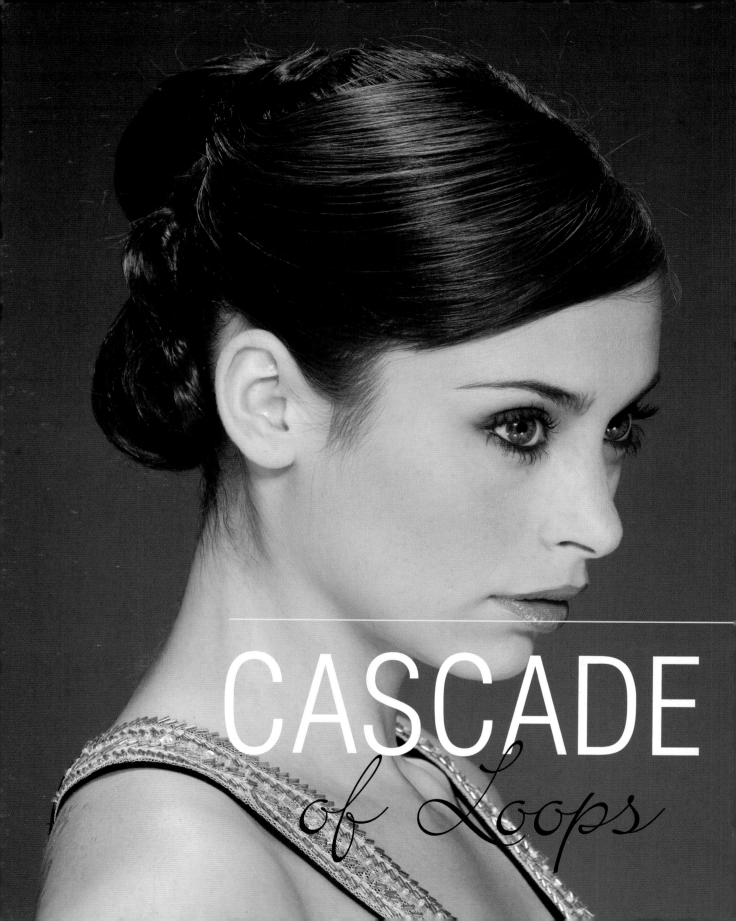

CASCADE
of Loops

54

With three central loops and several side loops, this design flows gently like a trickling forest stream.

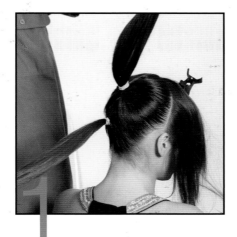

1. Wash and blow dry hair straight. Divide the hair into front and back sections with a part that extends from ear to ear over the crown. Hold the front hair in a clip. Divide the back hair into top and bottom sections with an upside-down V part. Gather each section in a ponytail. Draw a lock of hair in each ponytail, brush into a flat strip, and wrap around the base of the ponytail to conceal the elastic band.

2. Backcomb the bottom ponytail with a tail comb.

3. Mist with holding spray and blow dry to make a flat strip of hair.

4. Roll the hair downwards over a finger into a large loop. Secure the loop with bobby pins, leaving the ends loose.

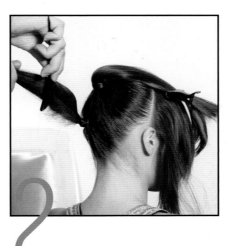

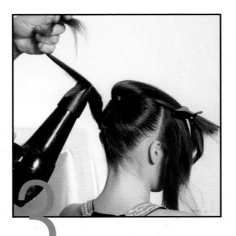

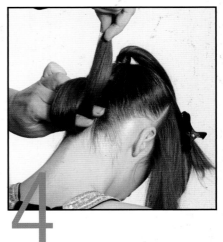

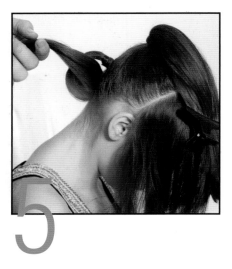

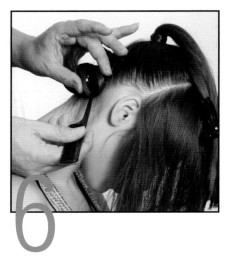

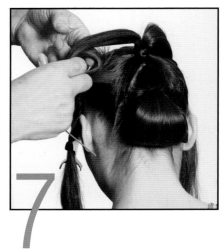

5. Brush the ends into a flat strip and draw upwards into the loop.

6. Coil the ends into a flat Figure 6 and secure with hair-pins at the nape of the neck on the right side of the loop.

7. Divide the top ponytail into two sections. Coil the left section into a flat Figure 6.

8. Draw the Figure 6 down-wards and to the left of the loop at the bottom of the head. Secure with hairpins.

9. Roll the right section of the top ponytail over a finger and into a loop. Secure with bobby pins just above the bottom ponytail, leaving the ends loose.

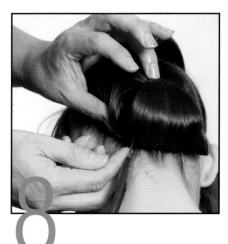

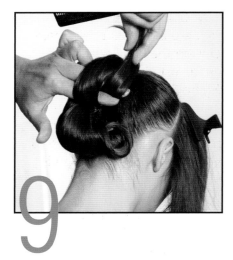

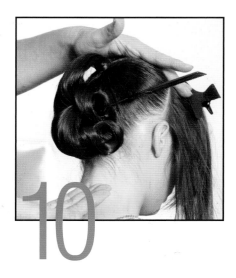

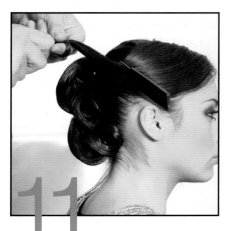

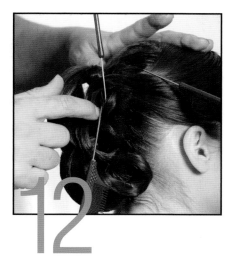

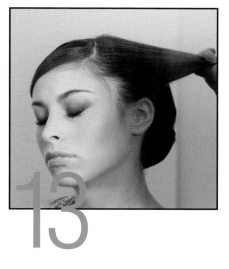

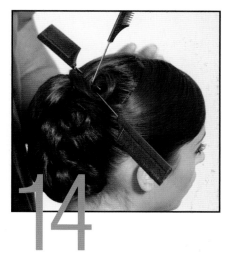

10. Coil the ends into a flat Figure 6 and secure with hairpins on the right side of the head, just above the other flat Figure 6.

11. Brush the front right hair backwards. Use a tail comb for support, then draw the ends upwards.

12. Coil into a flat Figure 6 beside the top loop, using tail combs for support.

13. Brush the front left hair backwards and draw over to the back of the head.

14. Wrap the hair into a circle using tail combs for support. Secure with hairpins on the right side of the head.

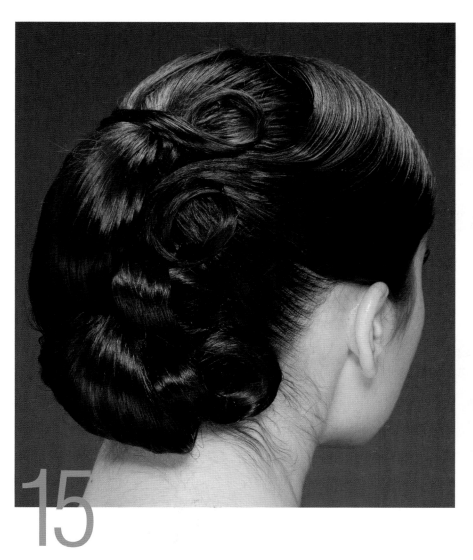

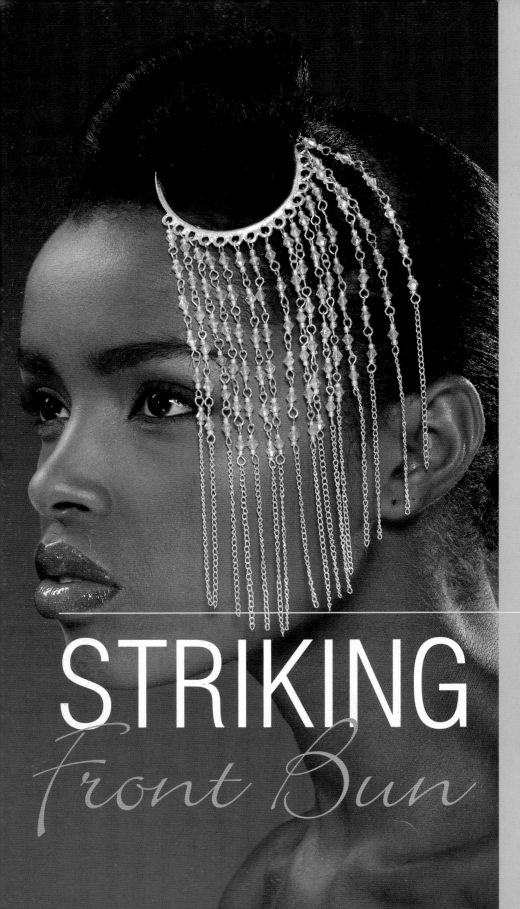

STRIKING
Front Bun

55

Show off a remarkable bracelet or round hair accessory with this design. The accessory is displayed over the face, so choose one that is really striking.

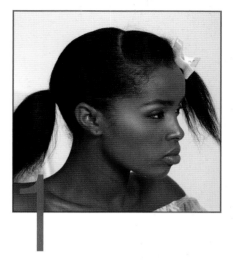

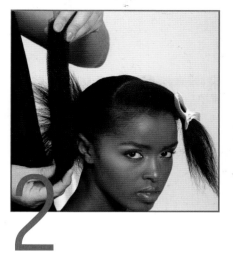

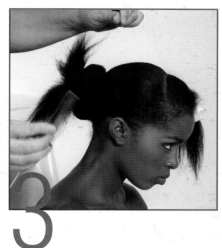

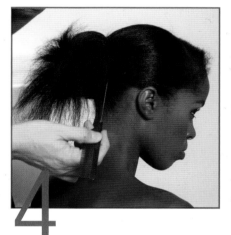

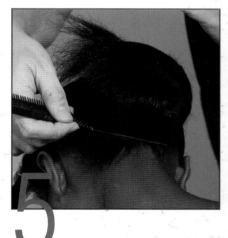

1. Wash and blow dry hair straight. Hold the bangs in a clip and gather the rest of the hair in a low ponytail.

2. Select a piece of sponge that is about 2 inches wide and 6 inches long.

3. Wrap the sponge around the ponytail and secure with a pin.

4. Brush the hair at the top of the ponytail upwards and over the sponge. Tuck the ends under the band towards the base of the ponytail.

5. Repeat all around the sponge, drawing the hair over the sponge and tucking it under on the other side.

6. Mist with holding spray and blow dry. Secure with hairpins all around.

7. Backcomb the bangs.

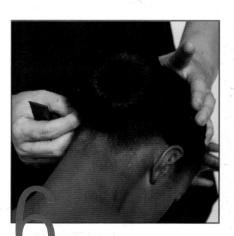

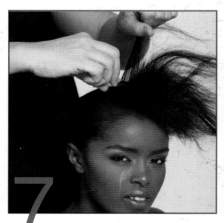

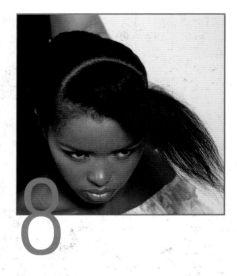

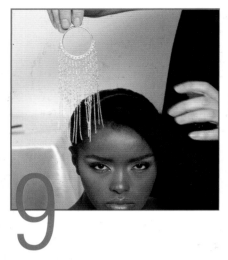

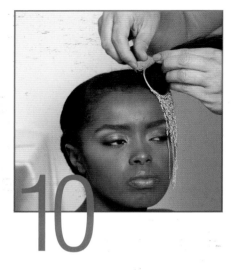

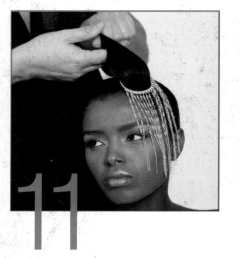

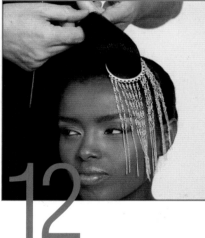

8. Brush the bangs forwards and secure with a seam of pins at the brow.

9. Select a round hair accessory or piece of jewelry.

10. Draw the accessory onto the bangs.

11. Brush the bangs upwards and over the top of the hair accessory.

12. Roll the bangs over a finger.

13. Form a high roll and secure with hairpins.

14. Mist with holding spray.

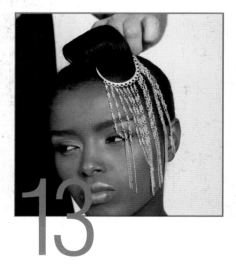

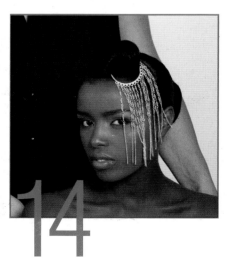

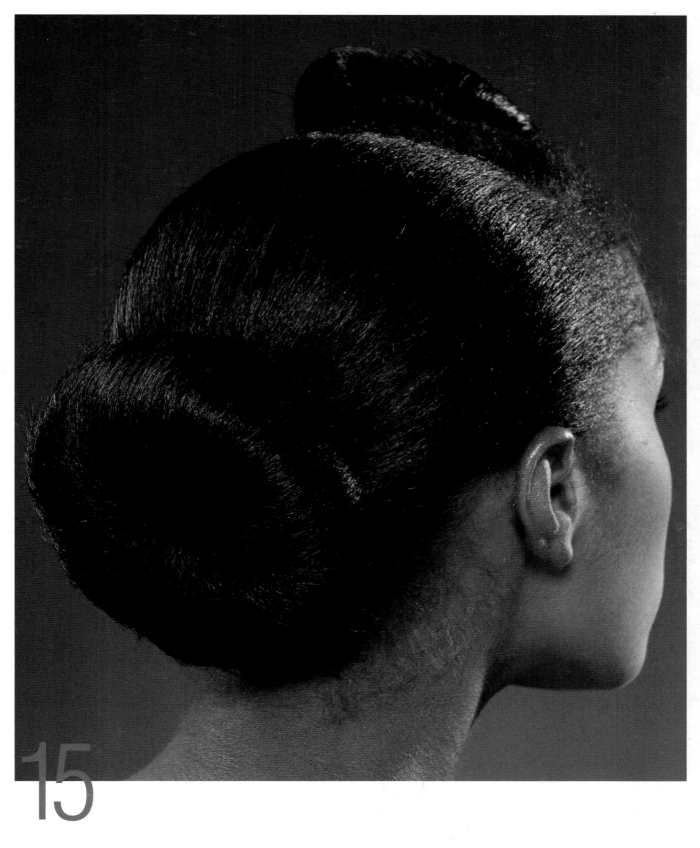

15

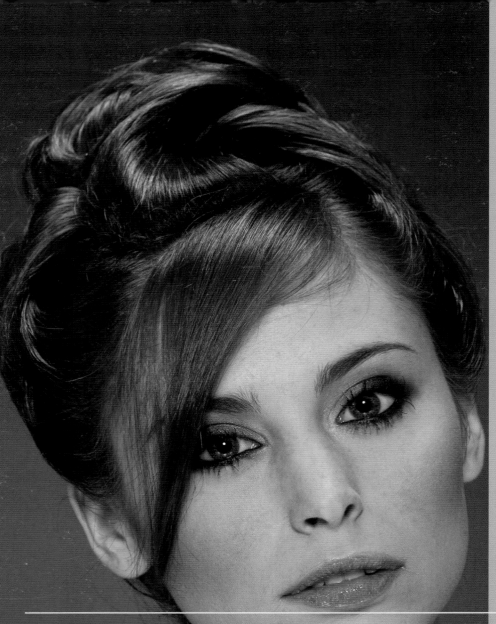

56

CORNUCOPIA
of Curls

With its assortment of curls and twirls, this is a perfect style for an elegant afternoon affair. Highlight the bare neck with a thick choker.

1. Wash and blow dry hair wavy. Backcomb a round section of hair at the crown.

2. Gather the backcombed hair in a high ponytail.

3. Draw a lock of hair from the ponytail and brush into a flat strip. Wrap the strip around the base of the ponytail to conceal the elastic band. Divide the ponytail into three sections.

4. Brush the front section into a flat strip and roll forwards over a finger to form a loop. Secure the loop with hairpins, leaving the ends loose.

5. Roll the ends over a finger to form another loop and secure behind the first loop, forming a double loop with this section of hair.

6. Brush another section into a flat strip and roll backwards over a finger to make a loop. Secure the loop with hairpins, leaving the ends loose. Roll the ends into a loop, forming a double loop.

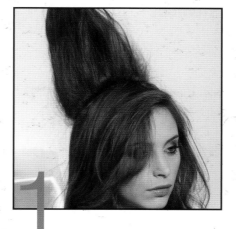

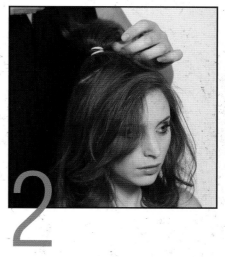

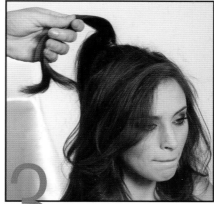

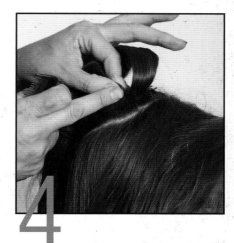

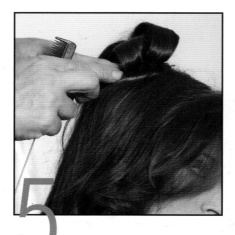

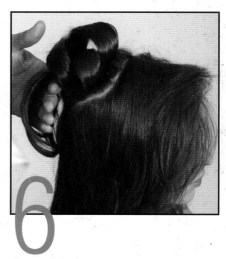

7. Repeat with the third section of hair, so that you have three double loops on the top of the head.

8. Gather a section of hair that extends from the loops to the bangs and brush into a flat strip.

9. Twist the hair upwards and backwards, towards the middle of the head. Make a double loop with the hair and secure it between two of loops.

10. Gather hair from a similar section to the right of the first section. Make a double loop and secure between two existing loops.

11. Repeat on the left side of the head, making a double loop that meets with the double loop from the right side.

12. Gather hair from a section behind the right ear and twist at the roots upwards. Secure between the loops at the top of the head, leaving the ends loose.

13. Repeat to make three more twisted sections of hair with the loose ends at the back of the head.

14. Mist the loose ends with holding spray and curve into arcs that wrap around the loops, using tail combs for support.

15. Secure with hairpins and remove the tail combs.

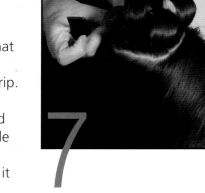

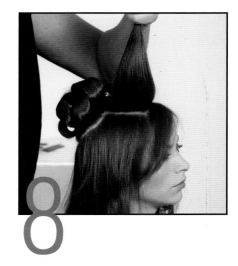

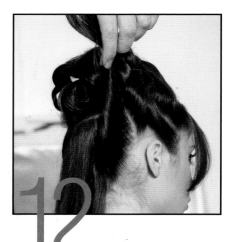

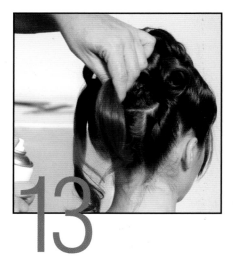

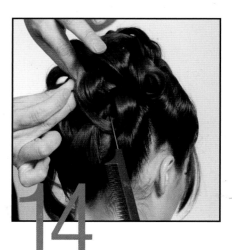

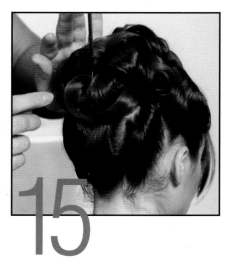

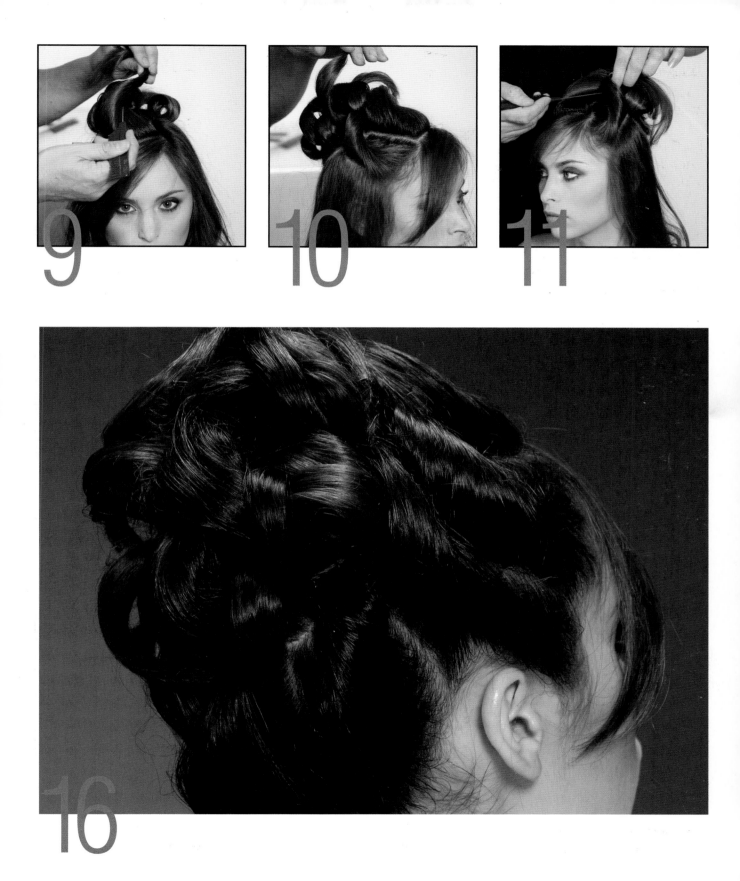

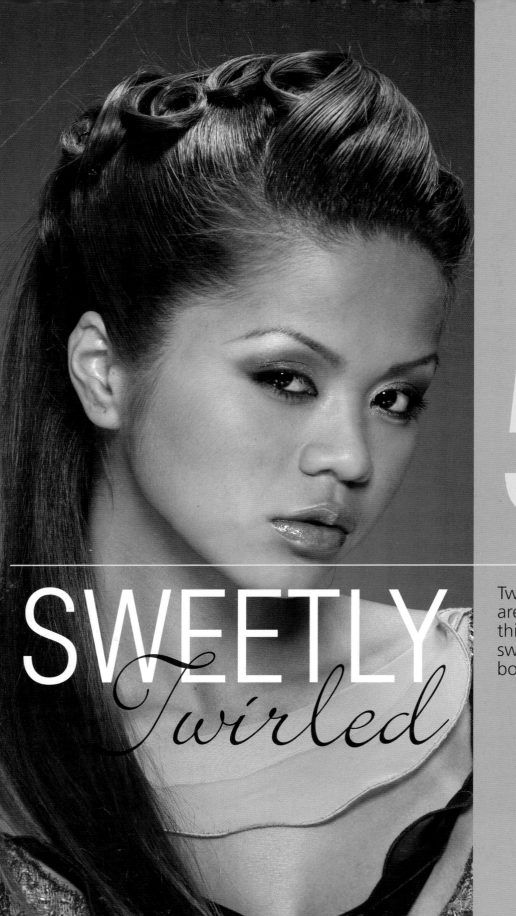

57

SWEETLY
Twirled

Two distinct designs are gently blended in this hairstyle. The top swirls gently and the bottom lies straight.

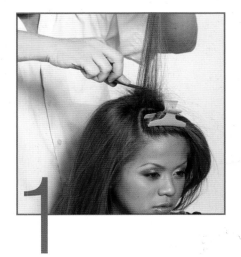

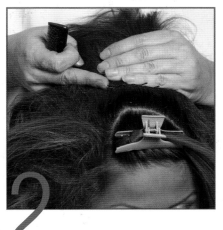

1. Wash and blow dry hair straight. Make a U-shaped part at the top of the head. Hold the hair in front of the part in a clip. Backcomb the hair behind the part.

2. Backcomb all of the hair behind the part.

3. Brush the hair in the middle of the head backwards and secure with bobby pins at the crown.

4. Brush back the hair at the left and right sides, making an arc-shaped seam of pins at the top of the head.

5. Brush the hair on the right side upwards, from the brow to the nape of the neck.

6. Secure with a seam of pins. Repeat on the left side.

7. Draw out a lock of hair from behind the seam of pins and brush into a flat strip.

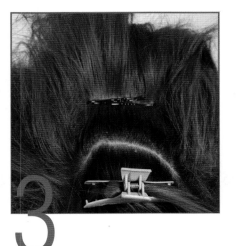

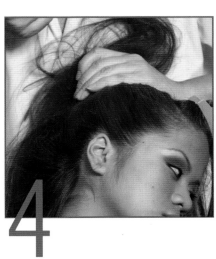

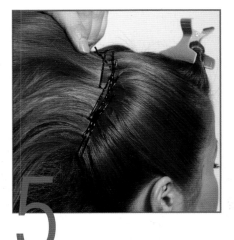

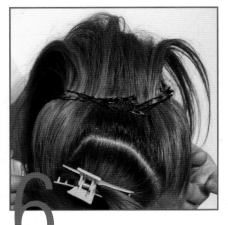

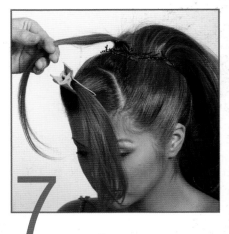

8. Wrap the hair into a circle by drawing it forwards and then backwards, using tail combs for support. Make an effort to conceal some of the pins with the circle.

9. Draw a section of hair to the right of the first section and brush into a flat strip. Draw towards the front of the head and loop backwards to create another circle of hair that conceals the pins.

10. Repeat to make a third circle that conceals the pins on this side of the head.

11. Divide the bangs into three sections. Brush a section backwards towards the seam of pins. Coil into a flat Figure 6 and secure near the seam of pins. Repeat with the other sections of hair, creating flat Figure 6s that conceal the seam of pins at the top.

12. Lift the hair and blow dry to add volume.

13. Draw a section of hair from the left side of the head and coil into a flat Figure 6 that conceals the seam of pins on this side.

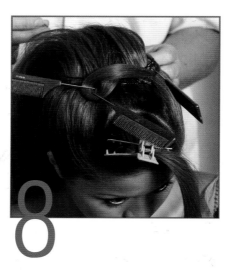

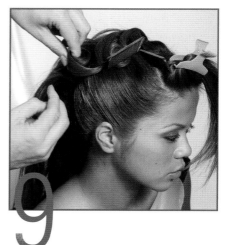

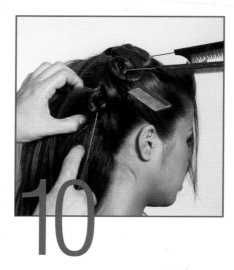

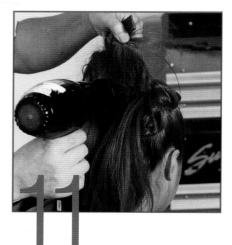

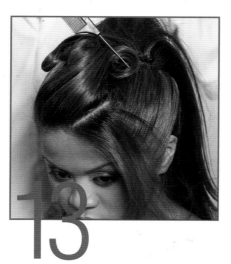

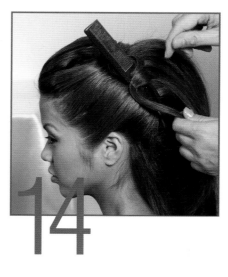

14. Repeat with another section of hair, coiling it into a flat Figure 6 behind this section.

15. Backcomb the hair in the middle of the head at the roots, working your way upwards from the neck to the crown. Mist with holding spray and blow dry on medium heat.

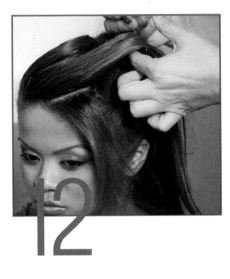

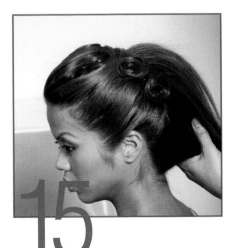

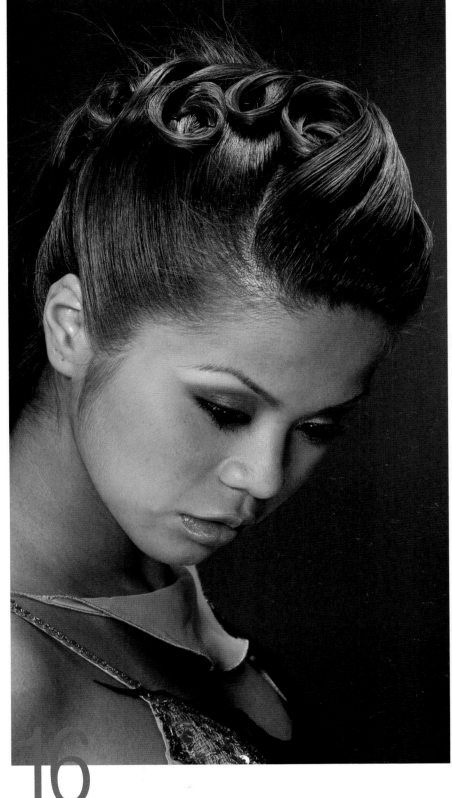

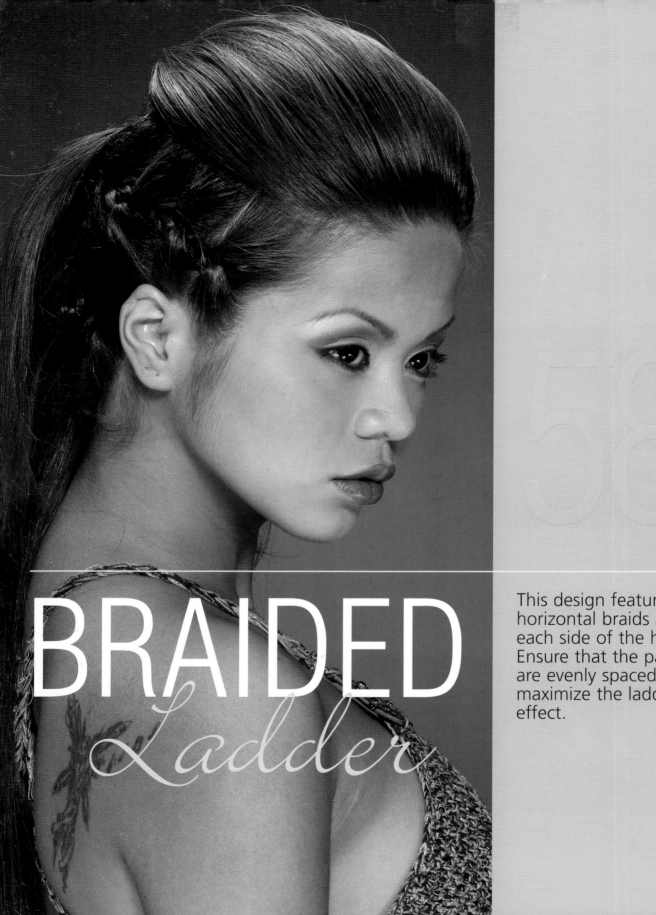

58

BRAIDED
Ladder

This design features horizontal braids along each side of the head. Ensure that the parts are evenly spaced to maximize the ladder effect.

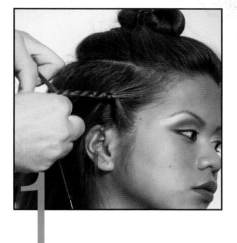

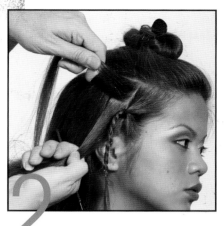

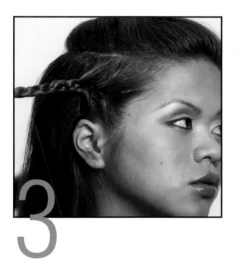

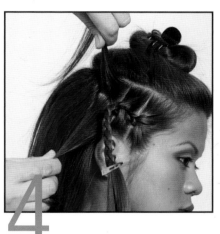

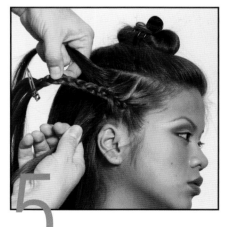

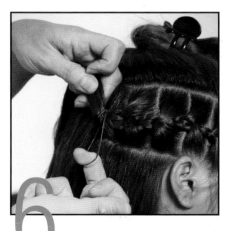

1. Wash and blow dry hair straight. Make right and left side parts that meet at the crown. Hold the hair above the parts in a clip. Make a vertical part on the right side of the head and divide into three sections. Mist with liquid spray and plait a braid that is about 2 inches long.

2. Make a vertical part behind the braid and divide the hair into top and bottom sections. Place the braid in the middle of these two sections.

3. Plait another braid, using these two sections and the braid.

4. Secure the braid temporarily with a clip. Make a vertical part behind the braid and divide the hair into top and bottom sections, placing the braid in the middle of these two sections.

5. Plait another braid, using these two sections and the braid.

6. Continue in this manner to make a horizontal braid that integrates five sections of hair. Secure with an elastic band close to the roots, leaving the ends loose.

7. Take a section of hair from behind the ear that runs from the braided area to the nape of the neck. Divide the hair into three sections and plait into a braid, leaving the ends loose.

8. Make a vertical part behind the braid and divide the hair into top and bottom sections. Place the braid between these two sections and plait a new braid. Continue in this manner to make a horizontal braid that integrates three sections of hair. Secure with an elastic band close to the roots, leaving the ends loose. Repeat to make similar braids on the right side of the head.

9. Release the hair at the top of the head and backcomb.

10. Mist with holding spray and brush backwards.

11. Secure with a seam of pins at the top of the head, so that the seam is in line with the ends of the braids.

12. Divide the loose ends from the top right braid into two sections. Draw one section over the back of the head, concealing the seam of pins. Secure on the left side with hairpins.

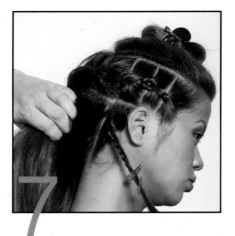

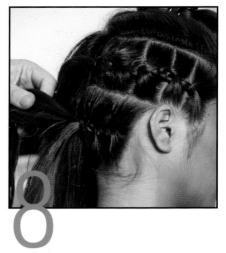

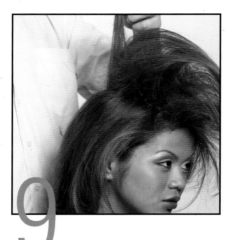

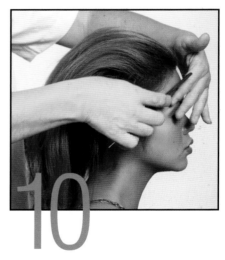

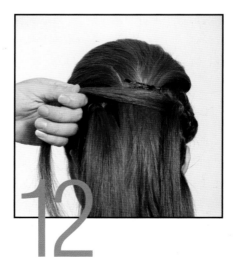

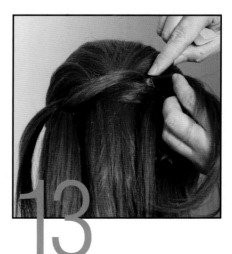

13. Repeat on the left side of the head, dividing the loose ends from the top braid into two sections and drawing the bottom section over the back of the head. Secure on the right side of the head with hairpins.

14. Arrange the loose ends at the back of the head so the look is symmetrical and neat.

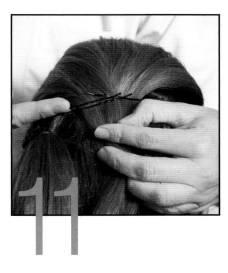

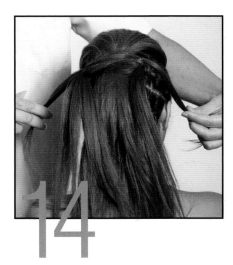

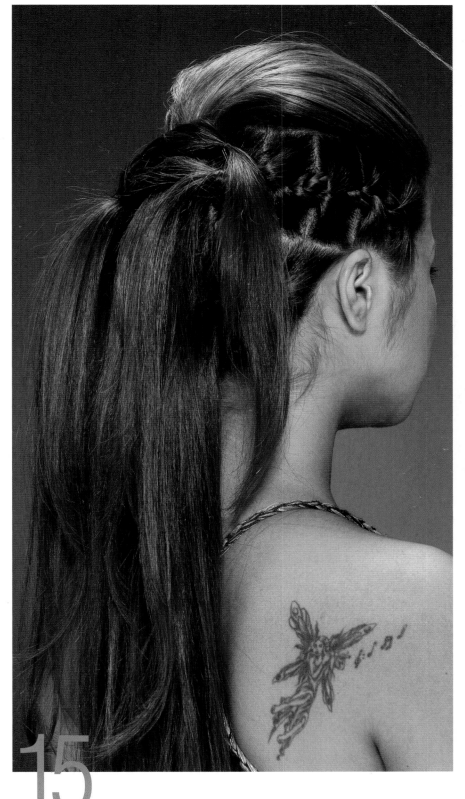

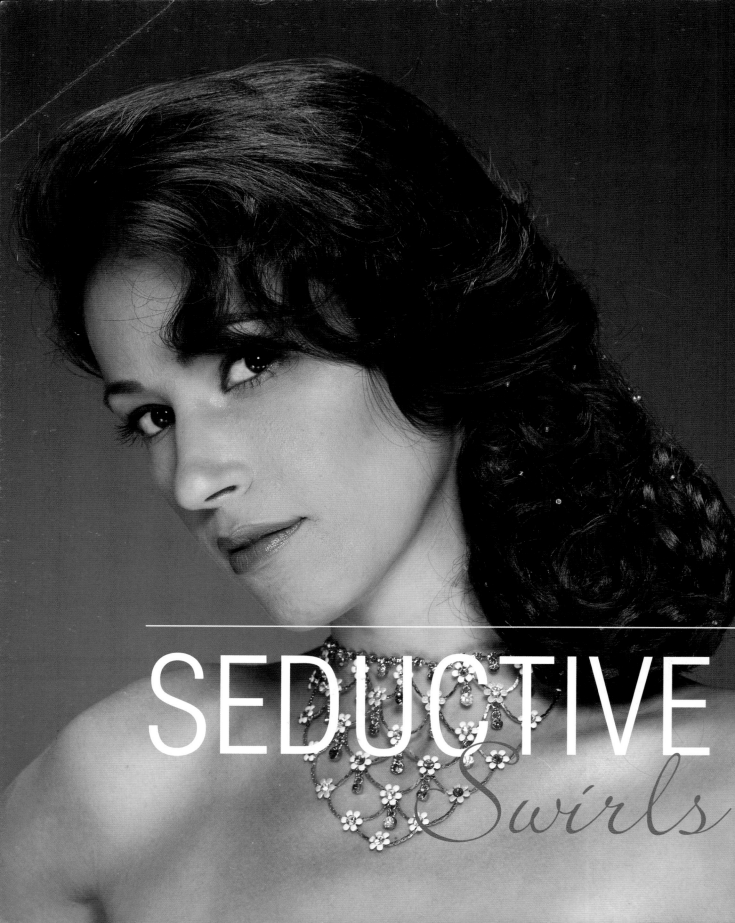

SEDUCTIVE *Swirls*

59

Gather the hair over the left shoulder to create a look that is soft yet sculpted. Choose a decorated hair accessory that matches your outfit.

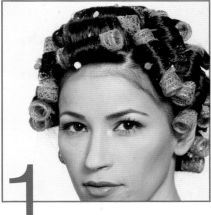

1. Massage strong styling mousse into the hair and set in rollers.

2. Blow dry hair then remove the rollers. Separate each curl into three locks of hair.

3. Make a U-shaped part that extends from the edge of each eyebrow over the crown. Hold the hair in front of the part in a clip. Draw the hair behind the part to the left side of the head.

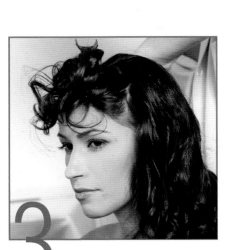

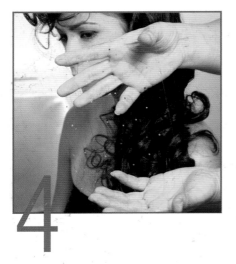

4

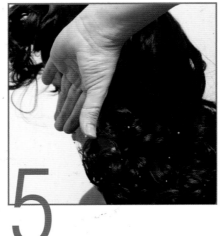

5

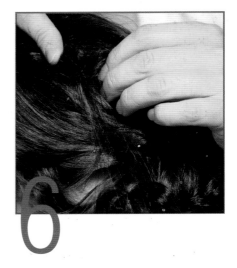

6

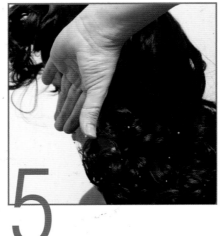

7

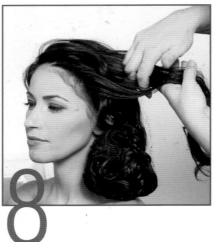

8

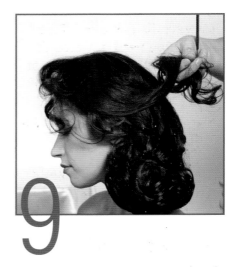

9

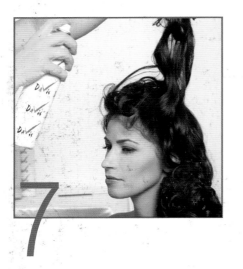

10

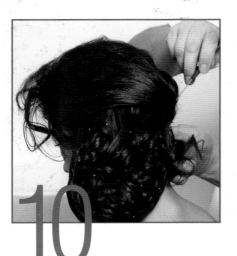

11

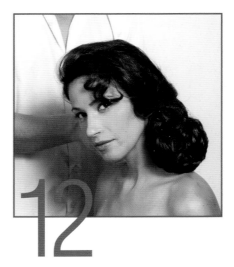

12

4. Select a hairnet, with or without beads, that is similar to the hair color.

5. Wrap the hairnet around the bottom of the hair.

6. Secure the hairnet with pins near the left ear.

7. Release the hair from the clip and mist with holding spray.

8. Comb through the hair with your fingers.

9. Draw the hair around the back of the head, towards the right side. Leave a few locks at the brow.

10. Draw the hair over the top of the hairnet.

11. Tuck the ends around the right side of the hairnet and secure with a bobby pin.

12. Arrange the locks on the brow.

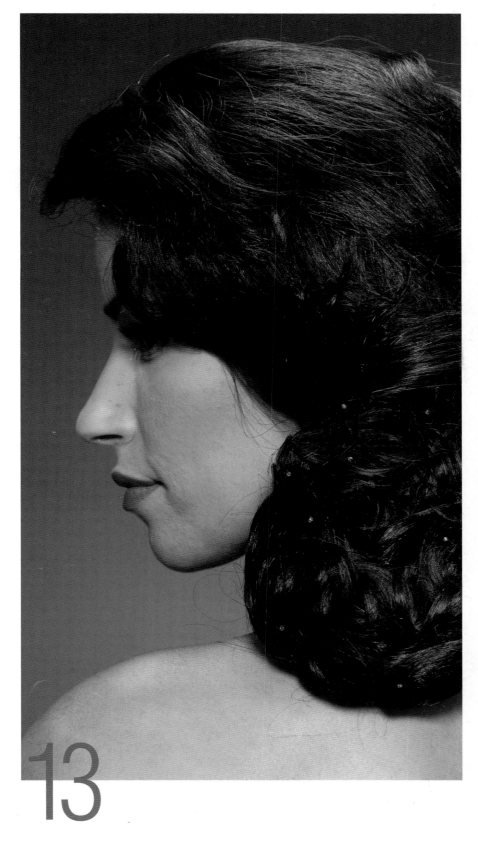

13

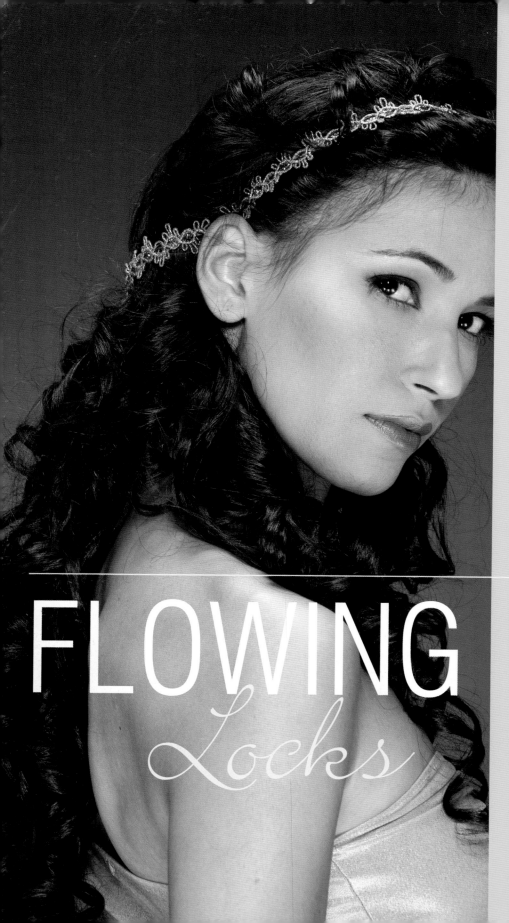

FLOWING
Locks

60

Few styles are quite as romantic as loosely flowing locks. This style includes an attractive ribbon that holds the hair away from the face, gathering it gently at the back.

1. Massage strong styling mousse into the hair and set in rollers.

2. Blow dry hair then remove the rollers one at a time, starting with the row along the nape of the neck.

3. Mist holding spray on each curl after it is unrolled.

4. Divide each curl into four or five locks.

5. Move up a level and release the next row of rollers.

6. Mist holding spray on each curl and divide into four or five locks.

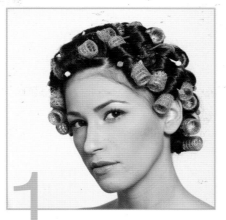

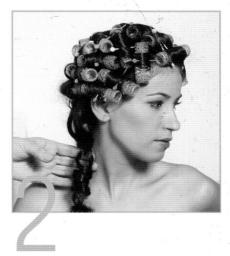

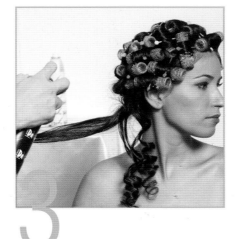

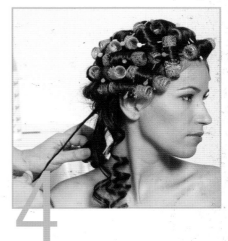

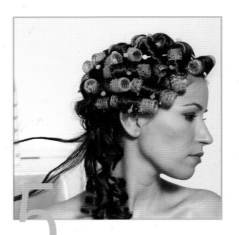

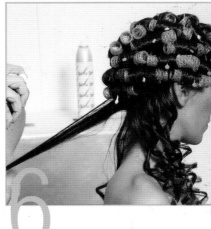

7. Continue in this manner, moving upwards towards the crown.

8. Divide each curl into four or five locks as you go.

9. Continue in this manner until you reach the roller at the brow.

10. For a carefree look, allow the hair to cascade down the back of the head.

11. For a gathered look, collect the hair loosely in a ribbon. Fold the ribbon in half, connecting the open ends to form a circle.

12. Draw the ribbon over the top of the head, so that it lies over the crown and horizontally across the back of the head.

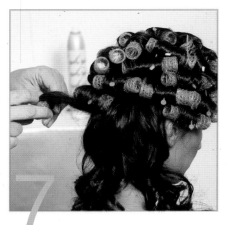

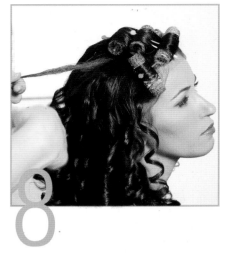

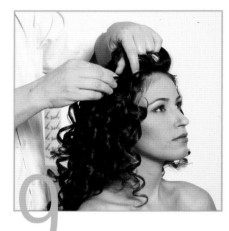

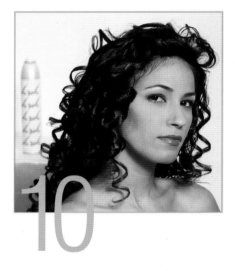

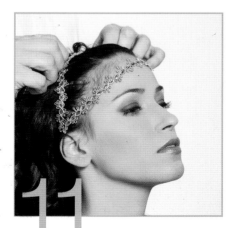

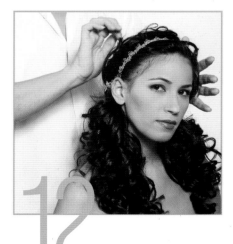

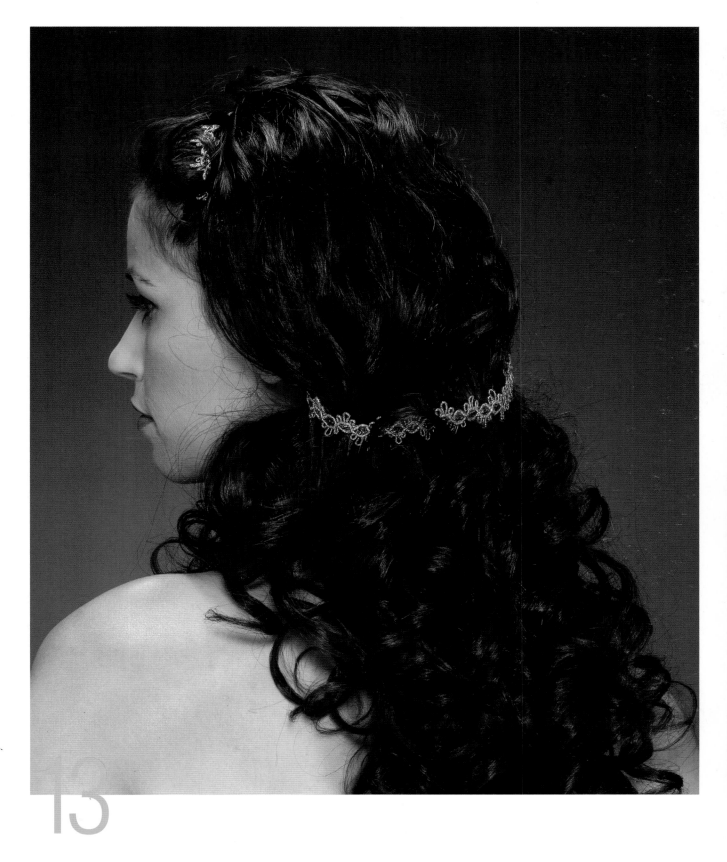

13

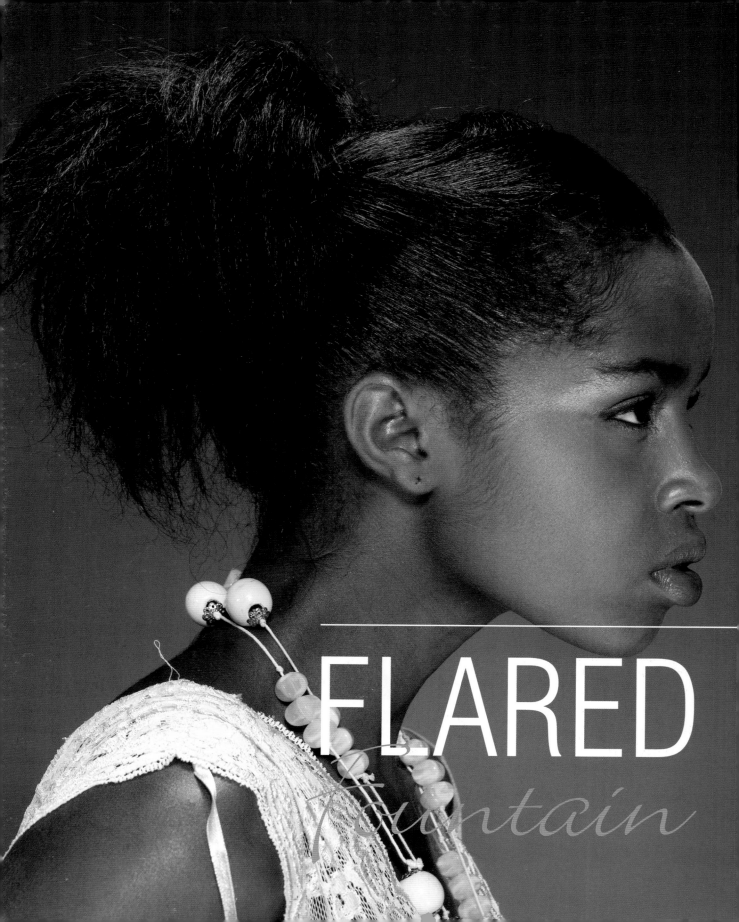

FLARED *Fountain*

61

The front of this design is woven and precise. The back features a fountain of hair that flows outwards in a stunning flare of hair.

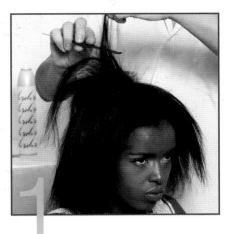

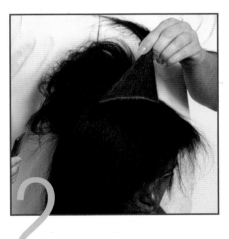

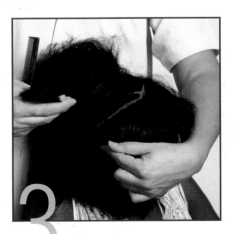

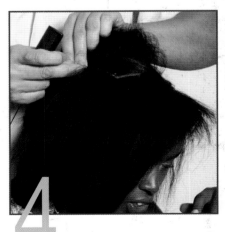

1. Wash and blow dry hair straight. Backcomb a section of hair at the top of the head to make a spongy base. Secure with a seam of pins.

2. Make a diagonal part on the right side of the spongy base. Brush the hair backwards and mist with holding spray. Draw the hair to the left, over the spongy base. Make a half-twist and secure with hairpins to the spongy base.

3. Make a diagonal part to the left of the previous part. Brush the hair backwards and mist with holding spray.

4. Draw the hair behind the spongy base and to the right. Secure with bobby pins.

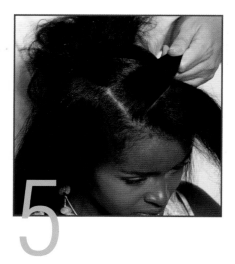

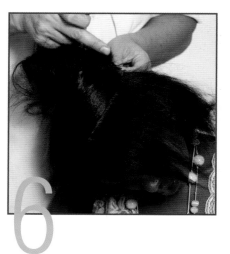

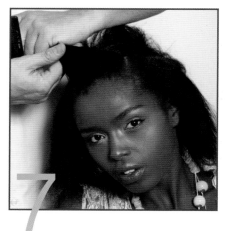

5. Make a part that extends from the top of the previous section to the brow. Mist with holding spray and draw backwards and to the left.

6. Draw the hair to the left of the spongy base and secure with bobby pins.

7. Mist the bangs with holding spray and draw backwards and to the right.

8. Secure with a bobby pin to the spongy base.

9. Mist the hair along the right side with holding spray and draw backwards and upwards.

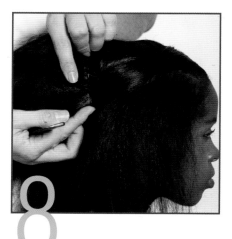

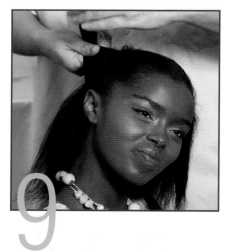

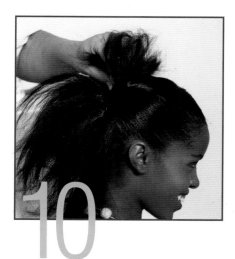

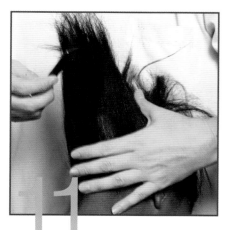

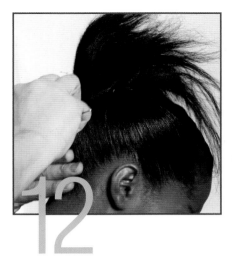

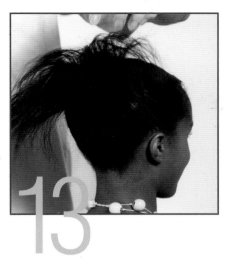

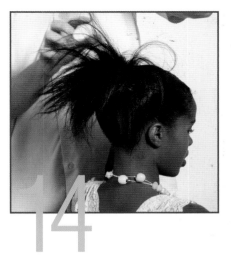

10. Make a half-twist and secure with bobby pins to the spongy base, leaving the ends loose.

11. Mist the loose hair at the back of the head with holding spray and brush upwards.

12. Secure with pins on the underside of the spongy base.

13. Massage styling cream into the loose ends at the top of the head.

14. Arrange the loose ends in a fountain of hair.

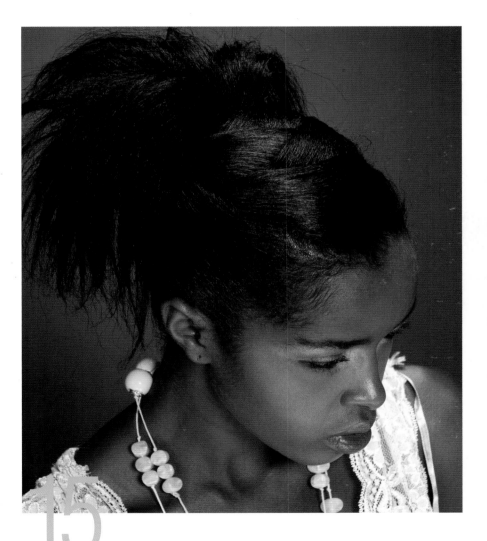

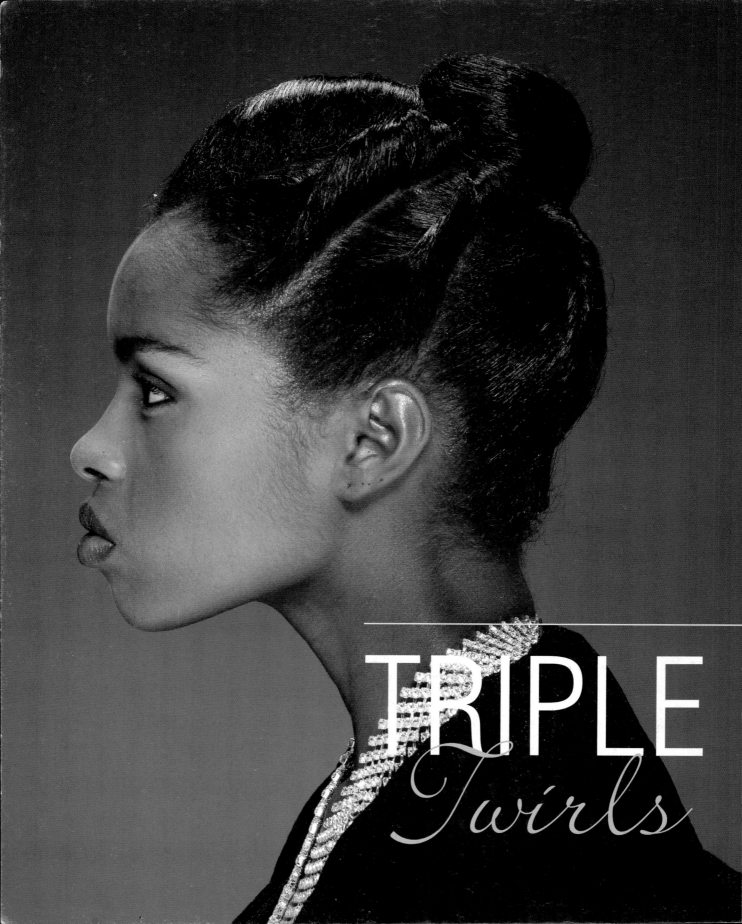

TRIPLE *Twirls*

62

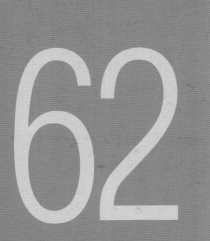

The lines in this design are clean and distinct. The twirls add a feminine softness. The combination is no less than riveting.

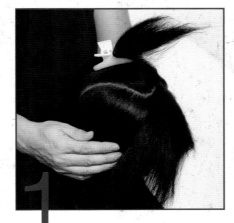

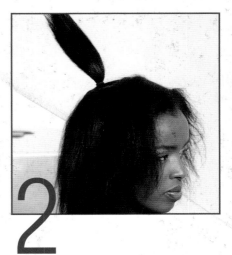

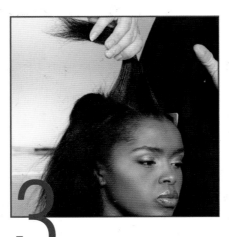

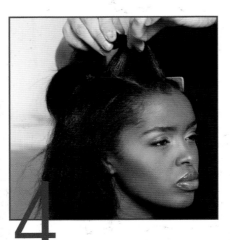

1. Wash and blow dry hair straight. Make a 2-inch-long rectangular part that extends from the crown towards the nape of the neck.

2. Gather the hair in this section in a high ponytail.

3. Gather hair from a rectangular section that extends from the brow to the ponytail. Mist with holding spray and brush upwards.

4. Grasp the ends of the hair with one hand and roll inwards. Stop rolling about 1 inch from the scalp. Mist with holding spray. Draw the ends of the hair in a half-twist towards the ponytail at the crown to make a standing roll.

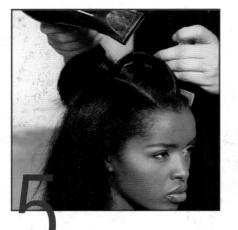

5

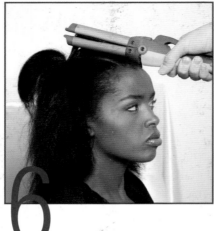

6

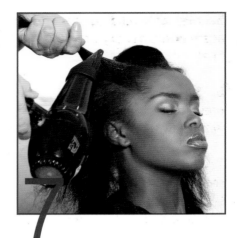

7

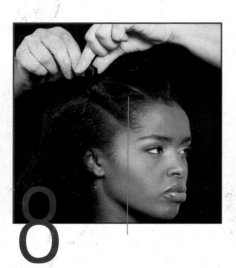

8

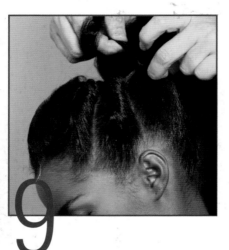

9

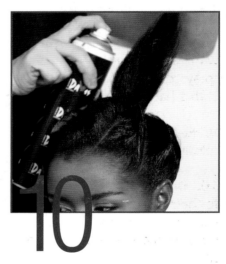

10

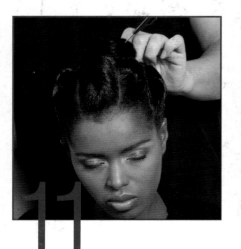

11

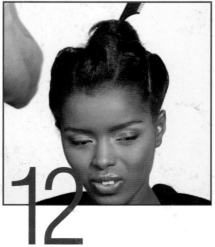

12

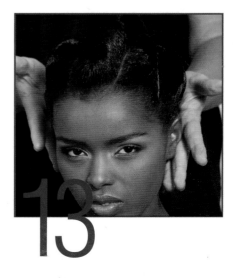

13

5. Mist with holding spray again and blow dry on medium heat.

6. Sharpen the angle by pressing the top of the roll with a hair straightener.

7. Gather hair from a similar section to the right of the first section. Mist with holding spray and brush upwards. Blow dry.

8. Roll the hair in a similar manner, so that the roll is about 1 inch from the scalp. Draw the ends of the hair in a half-twist towards the ponytail. Secure with hairpins, mist with holding spray, and sharpen the angle with a hair straightener.

9. Repeat to make standing rolls around the head.

10. Draw the ends of each roll to the ponytail at the back. Combine the hair in a large ponytail and mist with holding spray.

11. Using a tail comb for support, twist the hair around the ponytail.

12. Form a cone shape at the back of the head that conceals the base of the ponytail.

13. Mist generously with holding spray and blow dry.

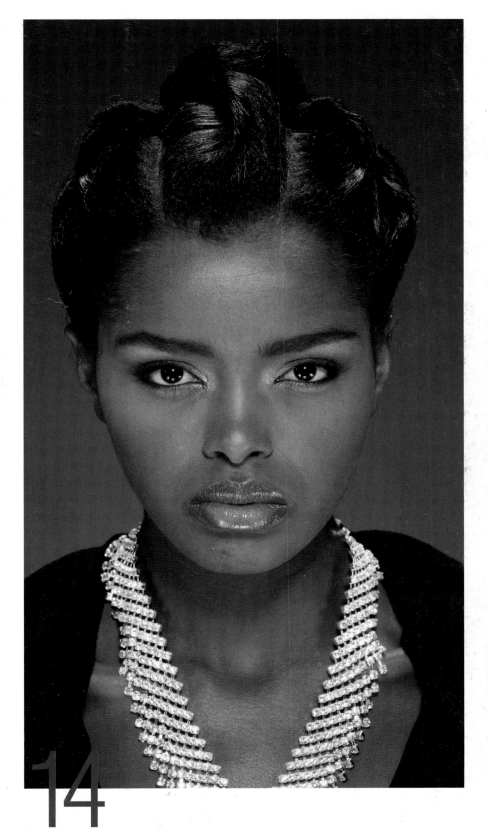

14

Index